Holistic Health Pathways:

Awaken Vitality and Resilience With Intentional Gratitude

Julius Torelli, MD

First Edition 2024

For Jessica and Daniel

My greatest teachers,

my most profound joy.

For you, I am grateful.

Contents

Introduction

Why Your Gratitude Journal May Not Be Working: The Power of Authentic Gratitude

The heart holds secrets no stethoscope can detect—a truth I discovered during my three decades as a cardiologist that shattered everything I learned in medical school.

By late 2006, after twenty years of practicing medicine, a pattern became apparent. Patients were coming into medical offices across the country - including mine - with symptoms but no physical findings. Despite thorough evaluations, we could find no physical cause for their headaches, abdominal pain, heart palpitations, and persistent fatigue. Their symptoms were 'medically unexplained.'

What initially appeared to be a frustrating gap in modern medicine gradually revealed itself as something far more profound. A window into an entirely different dimension of human health, where emotions and physical symptoms intertwined in a mysterious language that traditional medical training had never taught me to understand.

An Unexpected Awakening

It was a late Friday evening when I experienced something extraordinary in the most ordinary of places—my local grocery store.

Driving home exhausted from a grueling week and fighting a persistent depression that had plagued me, I just wanted to get home. I had no intention of leaving the house that weekend. But with an empty refrigerator waiting, I forced myself to stop.

Going grocery shopping is something I used to enjoy. Not these days, however, when there was little I enjoyed. Therapists called it depression. I called it misery.

All the therapists recommended medication, citing a "brain chemical imbalance" as the culprit. The medicines proved ineffective, their side effects alarming. One therapist suggested keeping a gratitude journal, backed by research showing its benefits for depression. I wrote faithfully for months, yet my emotional state remained unchanged.

I believed in practicing gratitude as an emotional aid. But how does one feel grateful when life keeps pounding you back into the canvas every time you try to get up? I felt like an amateur boxer in the rink against Mike Tyson, heavyweight champ.

Though I noticed little improvement at first, I persisted with the gratitude exercise beyond the journal entries. Over time, I observed the practice offered me a way to shift my perspective through finding just one small thing to appreciate in the moment. I noticed a difference between when I felt genuine gratitude versus the forced appreciation of an assigned journaling task. But this difference was nowhere near what I was about to experience.

Sitting in the grocery store parking lot, I searched for something genuine to appreciate. My fifteen-year-old Dodge Intrepid, with over two-hundred-fifty thousand miles, started reliably every morning. I was authentically grateful. I felt a slight lift.

I was grocery shopping, something I once enjoyed. Another moment of genuine appreciation. My spirits rose further. This seemed to give me strength, even a tinge of desire to get out of my car.

I walked into the grocery store. Standing in the produce section, holding a tomato, I experienced something I can't describe in words, something akin to witnessing the Northern Lights or standing at the Grand Canyon's edge. It was awe.

My chest, constricted for months, expanded fully as tears of gratitude welled up. This tomato was the culmination of natural processes, human cooperation, and countless hours of labor. I hadn't tilled soil, planted seeds, or tended crops. Yet here it was, ready to nourish me.

This awareness cascaded through every aisle. In the bread section, I marveled at dozens of varieties, each loaf representing an extensive, intricate journey from wheat field to shelf. I hadn't plowed the soil, harvested the crops, separated the kernels from the chaff, cleaned the grain, or milled the grain into flour. I thought about all the people involved: the farmers, the equipment operators, the truck drivers, the millers - and this was before the flour even became bread!

This realization extended beyond just bread. Every item on these shelves - whether produce, meat, or packaged goods - represented similarly complex networks of people and processes working in concert to stock our stores with food.

What began as a routine errand transformed into a profound lesson in authentic gratitude, as I finally grasped the massive collaborative effort behind even the simplest grocery store purchase.

Stepping out with my groceries, I absorbed the beautiful fall night. I was grateful. My car started. Grateful again. During the forty-five-minute drive home, I experienced an unfamiliar emotion. It wasn't happiness, contentment, excitement, or amazement—but peace. Peace for the first time in a long time. I noticed something else, a small smile on my face.

The Journey from Traditional to Holistic Medicine

The research findings, along with my transformative experience, reshaped my medical practice. This realization pushed me beyond traditional medical training to explore the broader dimensions of health—emotional, behavioral, mental, social, cultural, and spiritual. I began adding a "prescription" for gratitude practice to the standard guideline directed Western therapies my patients were already on, particularly focusing on those with medically unexplained symptoms. Their symptoms often improved. Their responses sometimes exceeded both of our expectations.

One striking example involved a woman with severe heart failure awaiting transplant. After adding a gratitude practice to her current medical regimen, her condition improved dramatically over six months. She progressed from struggling to walk one city block to completing two-mile walks. Eventually, she no longer needed a transplant.

Lesson 1

What is Gratitude?

Defining gratitude is challenging from my perspective. It's one of those things; you know it when you see it. Dictionary definitions could be more helpful and make more sense since they're circular. The Merriam-Webster definition of gratitude is "the state of being grateful," which is useless.

Gratitude encompasses an emotional state, a virtue, and a practice. Gratitude as an emotional state is when an individual recognizes and appreciates what they have in their life or the positive aspects of their experiences. It involves acknowledging the good things and expressing thankfulness for them, whether tangible (like a gift or a favor) or intangible (like the beauty of a sunrise or the love of a pet).

Gratitude as a virtue signifies the propensity to show thankfulness and return kindness. As a practice, it refers to regularly recognizing and expressing appreciation for the positive aspects of life.

It's important to note that gratitude is about acknowledging the big things in life and appreciating the small, everyday things that often go unnoticed. It involves a shift in perspective. The change is from focusing on what's wrong or lacking to acknowledging the already present abundance.

Research shows gratitude can have many benefits, including improved psychological health, better relationships, increased happiness, and reduced stress and depression. This is because practicing gratitude helps individuals focus on the positive aspects of life, which can increase feelings of contentment and satisfaction.

Understanding Gratitude

Gratitude is simply a feeling of appreciation. It's a sense of thankfulness for the blessings, big or small, that life offers us. It could be the joy of a warm cup of coffee on a chilly day, the kindness of a stranger, or the love of our friends and family. Gratitude encourages us to identify and cherish these moments of positivity in our lives.

The Benefits of Gratitude

Practicing gratitude yields a host of benefits, both psychological and physical. These include, but are not limited to:

1. **Increased Happiness:** Regularly expressing gratitude shifts our focus from what's wrong to what's right, leading to increased joy and happiness.

2. **Reduced Stress and Depression:** By focusing on the positive, we can reduce the symptoms of stress and depression.

3. **Improved Sleep:** Keeping a gratitude journal before bed can help with insomnia and improve overall sleep quality.

4. **Boosts Self-Esteem:** Gratitude helps us appreciate other people's accomplishments rather than feeling envious, increasing self-esteem.

5. **Fosters Resilience:** Regularly practicing gratitude helps us bounce back from stress and trauma.

The Science Behind Gratitude

The positive effects of gratitude aren't just anecdotal; science backs them. Research in positive psychology has shown that gratitude practices can activate the hypothalamus, a part of the brain responsible for several critical bodily functions, including stress levels and sleep patterns.

Gratitude also triggers the release of certain hormones and neurotransmitters, such as dopamine and serotonin. These neurotransmitters play critical roles in pleasure and regulating mood. As we progress in this book, we'll delve deeper into these scientific aspects.

A pivotal finding emerges from the research on gratitude: emotional depth matters more than routine practice. Studies show that participants who formed genuine emotional connections during gratitude exercises experienced significantly greater improvements in well-being compared to those who treated it as just another daily task.

Keep this principle of emotional engagement at the forefront as you explore the exercises in this book—it's the key to their transformative power. Approach each exercise with mindfulness and intention. I like to think of this method as "intentional gratitude." Keeping a gratitude journal is helpful but not required with this technique. You can engage in it at any moment. We will explore this flexible process throughout the book.

Overview

This 10-lesson book guides you in cultivating gratitude in your life. We'll journey together through understanding gratitude, its science, various gratitude practices, maintaining a gratitude journal, and overcoming challenges in practicing gratitude. We'll also discover how to extend gratitude to others and the concept of radical gratitude.

Exercise: Personal Reflection on Past Experiences of Gratitude

Now, let's dive into our first interactive exercise: personal reflection on experiences of gratitude. This exercise enables you to look back and identify moments when you felt a strong sense of gratitude.

Find a quiet, comfortable space and allow 10-15 minutes for this exercise. Close your eyes and reflect on when someone did something for you that made you feel deeply grateful. Whether it was a generous action or a minor act of kindness, bring up the feeling of that event and focus on how it made you feel.

Once you've spent time on this memory, open your eyes and write about your experience. Go deep with the experience. Describe the situation, the person involved, and the emotions you felt. The goal is to relive that genuine experience of gratefulness and kick-start your journey into gratitude.

This exercise has provided you with a glimpse into the understanding of gratitude and its many benefits. Remember, the journey of gratitude is not about a destination, but the steps you take along the way. I look forward to seeing you in our next lesson, where we'll explore the science of gratitude.

Happy reflecting!

Lesson 2

The Science of Gratitude

Unraveling the Physical and Mental Health Benefits

Gratitude is a warm feeling of thankfulness towards the world or specific individuals. It's not just about acknowledging good in life, but also about recognizing where that goodness comes from. However, gratitude is more than just an emotional response; it's also a positive habit that individuals can cultivate to improve their quality of life.

Over the past two decades, many studies have shown the surprising life improvements that can stem from gratitude. Understanding the science behind these benefits and integrating gratitude into daily life can provide a practical pathway to improved mental and physical health and overall well-being.

The Science of Gratitude

Scientifically speaking, gratitude is not just an action. It is also a positive emotion that serves a biological purpose. Positive psychology and neuroscience have shown that expressing gratitude provides several psychological and physiological benefits. For instance, when we express gratitude, our brain releases dopamine and serotonin, two crucial neurotransmitters responsible for our emotions. They enhance our mood immediately, making us feel happier.

The Neuroscience of Gratitude

The profound effects of gratitude on our overall well-being are deeply rooted in our brains. Understanding the neuroscience behind gratitude can shed light on why it's such a powerful tool for enhancing mental health and well-being.

1. **Dopamine and the Reward System:** Dopamine, often known as the 'feel-good' neurotransmitter, plays a crucial role in our brain's reward system. When we express gratitude or receive thanks, our brain releases dopamine. This release triggers positive emotions, satisfaction, and pleasure. Essentially, our brain reinforces and encourages us to repeat behaviors associated with these positive feelings. So, when we practice gratitude regularly, we strengthen the neural pathways that stimulate dopamine production, effectively training our brains to feel happier and more content.

2. **Serotonin and Mood Regulation:** Serotonin, another key neurotransmitter, is often called the 'happy chemical' because it contributes significantly to happiness and well-being. It helps regulate our mood, sleep, appetite, and cognitive functions, including memory and learning. Research suggests that thinking about things we're grateful for boosts serotonin production in a region of the brain associated with emotional processing. This suggests that gratitude practice can be a natural way to increase serotonin levels, thus enhancing mood and combating depression and anxiety.

3. **Oxytocin and Social Bonding:** When we experience positive social interactions, including expressing or receiving gratitude, our bodies release oxytocin, often known as the 'love hormone' or 'social bonding hormone.' It enhances our sense of trust, empathy, and connectedness to others. Therefore, gratitude can

foster stronger relationships and social bonds, contributing to our overall sense of belonging and well-being.

4. **Brain Plasticity and the Gratitude Habit:** Importantly, our brains have a quality known as 'neuroplasticity' - the ability to form new neural pathways based on experience. This means that gratitude can change the brain's neural structures with consistent practice, making it more efficient at recognizing and appreciating the good in life.

In summary, the neuroscience of gratitude provides a fascinating insight into how this simple practice can significantly improve our physical and mental well-being. It reinforces that gratitude isn't merely a societal virtue but a critical tool to help us lead happier, healthier, and more fulfilling lives.

The Benefits of Gratitude on Mental Health

Gratitude can significantly improve psychological health and well-being. Acknowledging and appreciating what we have can shift our thinking from negativity and complaints to positivity and contentment. Psychological benefits associated with gratitude include:

1. **Increased Happiness and Positive Emotion:** Gratitude is strongly associated with greater happiness. It helps people feel positive emotions, savor pleasant experiences, and build strong relationships. According to a study published in the *Journal of Personality and Social Psychology*, a gratitude journal can increase long-term well-being by over 10 percent.

   Gratitude helps us focus on the positive aspects of our lives, which increases positive emotions like joy, love, and contentment.

Research has consistently found that people who regularly practice gratitude report experiencing more positive emotions. According to research, people who regularly practice gratitude report higher levels of happiness. A study published in the *Journal of Personality and Social Psychology* found that participants who wrote about things they were grateful for were more optimistic and felt better about their lives.

2. **Reduced Negative Emotions and Depression:** Depression is a common mental disorder characterized by persistent sadness, a lack of interest in activities, and a decrease in the ability to function at work and home. Gratitude, emphasizing recognizing and appreciating the positive aspects of life, can play a crucial role in combating depression and fostering mental wellness. Gratitude can reduce many toxic emotions, from envy and resentment to frustration and regret. Robert Emmons, a leading researcher in the field of gratitude, has conducted multiple studies on gratitude and found that it significantly reduces symptoms of depression. Gratitude can encourage us to take better care of our physical health, which has beneficial effects on depression. Physical activity can boost mood and act as a natural antidepressant.

Research has shown a significant inverse relationship between gratitude and depression. A study published in the Journal of Counseling Psychology found that higher levels of gratitude predicted lower levels of depression. Another study published in the Clinical Psychology Review found that gratitude interventions effectively reduce depression among clinical populations.

3. **Enhanced Empathy and Reduces Aggression:** Grateful people are more likely to behave prosocially, even when others behave less kindly. A 2012 study by the University of Kentucky found that gratitude participants experienced more sensitivity and empathy towards others and decreased desire to seek revenge.

4. **Enhanced Self-Esteem:** Self-esteem refers to the overall subjective emotional evaluation of one's worth. It's a critical component of mental health and well-being. Gratitude, with its focus on appreciating the positive aspects of life and acknowledging the contributions of others, can significantly enhance self-esteem. Here's how gratitude contributes to improved self-esteem:

    • **Reducing Social Comparisons:** Gratitude allows us to appreciate other people's accomplishments without feeling inadequate or resentful. Focusing on gratitude makes us less likely to fall into the trap of unfavorable social comparisons, which can lead to negative self-evaluations and lower self-esteem. Instead, we appreciate the accomplishments and qualities of others, which can inspire us to pursue self-improvement without diminishing our self-worth.

    • **Promoting Positive Emotions:** The positive emotions associated with gratitude, such as joy, love, and contentment, can enhance our self-worth and confidence. When we feel good about life, those feelings often extend to how we feel about ourselves.

    • **Fostering Optimism:** Gratitude can foster a more optimistic outlook on life, which is closely linked to higher self-esteem. By recognizing and appreciating the positive aspects of our lives, we can maintain a more optimistic view of our future, which boosts self-confidence and self-esteem.

- **Building Relationships:** Gratitude can strengthen relationships, which can boost self-esteem. Positive social interactions and a sense of belonging can enhance our self-image and self-worth.

Research supports the connection between gratitude and self-esteem. A study published in the *Journal of Applied Sport Psychology* found that athletes who expressed higher levels of gratitude had higher self-esteem than those who expressed less gratitude. Another study in the Journal of Happiness Studies found a significant positive relationship between gratitude and self-esteem in university students. A 2014 study published in the *Journal of Applied Sport Psychology* found that gratitude increased athletes' self-esteem, an essential component of optimal performance. Other studies have shown that gratitude reduces social comparisons, enabling us to appreciate other people's accomplishments rather than feeling inadequate or resentful.

Cultivating gratitude can be a powerful way to boost self-esteem, enhancing our overall mental health and well-being.

5. **Improved Resilience:** Resilience is the ability to bounce back from stressful or traumatic events. It involves maintaining flexibility and balance when dealing with stressful circumstances and traumatic events. It's not about avoiding stress, but learning to thrive within it.

Gratitude plays a crucial role in enhancing resilience. By acknowledging the good things in life and recognizing the contributions of others, we develop a more positive outlook, which can help us deal with stress and adversity. Some ways gratitude contributes to resilience are:

- **Positive Reappraisal:** Gratitude can help us reframe our experiences more positively. Rather than focusing on what's going wrong, gratitude encourages us to appreciate what's going well. This positive reappraisal helps us manage stress and adversity by shifting our focus from adverse events to positive ones.

- **Building Positive Emotions:** According to psychologist Barbara Fredrickson's broaden-and-build theory of positive emotions, positive emotions broaden our awareness and encourage novel, varied, and exploratory thoughts and actions. Over time, this broadened behavioral repertoire builds skills and resources. By cultivating positive emotions like gratitude, we can develop our psychological resilience and resources, helping us bounce back from adversity.

- **Strengthening Relationships:** Gratitude can enhance our relationships by promoting positive interactions and mutual appreciation. Strong social connections are a vital component of resilience, providing emotional support and practical help in times of stress. We can strengthen these crucial social bonds by expressing gratitude to the people in our lives.

- **Cultivating an Attitude of Growth:** Gratitude can help us appreciate the lessons that come

- **With adversity.** By recognizing the potential for growth in our challenges, we can foster a growth mindset - another critical aspect of resilience.

Research supports the role of gratitude in enhancing resilience. For instance, a study published in the *Journal of Personality and Social Psychology* found that gratitude was a significant predictor of resilience following the September 11th terrorist attacks. Another study in the *Journal of Positive Psychology* found that gratitude predicted greater resilience in breast cancer patients.

Research also shows that gratitude reduces stress and plays a significant role in overcoming trauma. A 2006 study published in *Behavior Research and Therapy* found that Vietnam War Veterans with higher levels of gratitude experienced lower rates of Post-Traumatic Stress Disorder.

6. **Promotes Mental Strength:** Mental strength refers to an individual's resilience and fortitude to navigate challenges and bounce back from adversity. It involves emotional intelligence, self-regulation, and a positive mindset. Gratitude plays a significant role in enhancing mental strength, bolstering our ability to confront the challenges life throws our way. For years, research has shown gratitude reduces stress and plays a significant role in overcoming trauma and enhancing mental strength. Here are some ways in which gratitude contributes to mental strength:

- **Enhancing Emotional Well-being:** Gratitude boosts our mood and overall emotional well-being, which is critical for mental strength. It allows us to experience more positive emotions and helps reduce negative emotions like anger, fear, and resentment.

- **Promoting Optimism:** Gratitude fosters a more optimistic outlook on life, helping us to maintain a positive attitude even in the face of challenges. This optimism is crucial for mental strength as it encourages us to persist in facing obstacles and view these challenges as opportunities for growth, rather than insurmountable problems.

- **Reducing Stress:** Gratitude has been shown to reduce stress, a factor that can undermine mental strength. By focusing on what we're thankful for, we can manage our stress levels more effectively, fostering greater mental strength.

- **Encouraging Self-Improvement:** By appreciating what we have, we can also see the areas in our lives where we'd like to improve. This motivation for self-improvement and personal growth is essential to mental strength.

Cultivating gratitude in our daily lives can significantly enhance our mental strength, empowering us to face life's challenges with courage and resilience.

From a mental health perspective, gratitude can play a significant role. Studies by Dr. Robert Emmons have shown that gratitude effectively increases happiness and reduces depression.

Gratitude practices demonstrably reduce pain, stress, and depression in participants. They also report more happiness and joy, as well as experiencing lower symptoms of burnout. For example, maintaining a gratitude diary helps shift focus from what's wrong in our lives to what's going well, reducing the focus on distressing thoughts.

Integrating gratitude into daily life can be as simple as writing in a gratitude journal, writing thank-you notes, or mentally acknowledging what you are grateful for at the start or end of each day. By incorporating gratitude into our daily routine, we can improve our psychological well-being and overall quality of life.

Benefits of Gratitude on Physical Health

The physiological benefits of gratitude are just as impressive as the psychological ones. Gratitude has been shown to influence the body in multiple ways, from our sleep to our heart health. Let's delve into the science behind these benefits:

1. **Improved Sleep:** Research has consistently shown a link between gratitude and better sleep. In a study published in the *Journal of Psychosomatic Research*, individuals who wrote in a gratitude journal for 15 minutes before bed had a better sleep duration and quality than those who did not. This effect is likely because of the shift in focus from worries and negative thoughts to positive ones, which can facilitate a more restful state conducive to sleep.

2. **Reduced Levels of Pain:** Expressing gratitude can also help reduce pain levels. A Critical Care Nurse Journal study found that patients who maintained a gratitude journal reported reduced pain and stress levels. Gratitude might influence pain perception by shifting attention away from negative or painful thoughts and feelings.

3. **Lower Blood Pressure:** Regular expression of gratitude is also linked to lower blood pressure. According to research published in the *American Journal of Cardiology*, heart failure patients who kept gratitude journals for eight weeks showed reductions in inflammatory biomarkers and improved heart rate variability, a key indicator of reduced cardiac risk.

4. **Enhanced Immune Function:** Gratitude has been found to boost the immune system. Positive emotions, like gratitude, can enhance the production of immune-boosting natural killer cells. A study conducted at the Universities of Utah and Kentucky observed that stressed-out law students who were optimistic had more disease-fighting cells in their bodies.

5. **Improved Digestion:** While more research is needed, some studies suggest that positive emotions, including gratitude, may help improve digestion. Stress and negative emotions can disrupt the gut-brain axis, leading to issues like irritable bowel syndrome and other gastrointestinal disorders. Practicing gratitude promotes a more relaxed state, reducing stress, which may help improve digestion.

6. **Longer Lifespan:** While it's hard to prove definitively, some researchers believe that the cumulative effects of gratitude—better sleep, less stress, lower blood pressure, etc.—might contribute to a longer lifespan.

People who consciously count their blessings are less prone to physical illness. They experience fewer aches and pains and report feeling healthier than other people, according to a 2015 study published in the *Journal of Religion and Health*. But why is this the case?

One reason is that grateful people take better care of their health. They exercise more often and are more likely to attend regular check-ups, contributing to further longevity. This was demonstrated in a study in the journal *Personality and Individual Differences*, which found a direct link between gratitude and self-care behaviors.

By maintaining a gratitude journal and noting down the aspects of life for which you are grateful, you can increase your awareness of personal well-being, which may motivate one to take better care of their physical health.

Another intriguing link between gratitude and physical health is the impact on sleep. Researchers in *Applied Psychology: Health and Well-Being* found that writing in a gratitude journal improves sleep. Participants who spent just 15 minutes jotting down grateful sentiments before bed were found to sleep better and longer. This practice can be easily integrated into a bedtime routine.

Gratitude has a profound impact on our physiology. It's not just about feeling good; it's about promoting healthier bodies and longer, more fulfilling lives. By understanding these benefits, we can appreciate the importance of incorporating gratitude into our daily lives.

The Broader Benefits of Gratitude

Gratitude profoundly affects our physiology and psychology, promoting healthier bodies and more fulfilling lives. Beyond enhancing our physical and mental health, gratitude can provide many broader benefits that permeate every aspect of our lives. It can help us navigate personal relationships, professional interactions, and life perspectives. Here are some of the broader benefits of gratitude:

The Broader Benefits of Gratitude

Gratitude profoundly affects our physiology and psychology, promoting healthier bodies and more fulfilling lives. Beyond enhancing our physical and mental health, gratitude can provide many broader benefits that permeate every aspect of our lives. It can help us navigate personal relationships, professional interactions, and life perspectives. Here are some of the broader benefits of gratitude:

1. **Enhanced Empathy and Reduced Aggression:** Grateful people are more likely to behave in a pro-social manner, even when others behave less kindly. Gratitude encourages empathy and understanding, reducing our tendency to react aggressively or indifferently.

2. **Better Sleep:** Practicing gratitude can improve sleep quality. Reflecting on what we're grateful for can induce relaxation, helping us fall asleep faster and sleep more soundly.

3. **Career Benefits:** In the professional realm, gratitude can lead to better decision-making, increased productivity, and reduced stress and burnout. It can also foster a positive workplace environment, enhancing teamwork and collaboration.

4. **Academic Success:** For students, gratitude can improve academic performance. A positive outlook can enhance learning and motivation, leading to better grades and increased goal achievement.

5. **Promotes Altruism:** Gratitude can make us more altruistic. The more we recognize the kindness and generosity of others towards us, the more likely we are to pay it forward and act generously towards others.

6. **Fosters a Sense of Belonging and Community:** Gratitude fosters a sense of community by helping us recognize and appreciate our interconnectedness. It encourages a sense of belonging and mutual support, contributing to more robust, cohesive communities.

The benefits of gratitude extend far beyond ourselves. It's a powerful tool for fostering positive relationships, creating harmonious communities, and promoting a more caring and compassionate society.

A 2010 Journal of Personality and Social Psychology study found that gratitude triggers a positive relationship feedback loop. Expressing gratitude to a partner makes them feel positively acknowledged and strengthens the relationship bond. These feelings of gratitude can make people more willing to work through issues and less likely to retaliate against negative behavior.

In the professional world, gratitude can boost career success. In a work environment, showing appreciation can increase job satisfaction, reduce stress, and improve overall performance.

Gratitude has been found to increase mental strength, reduce materialistic attitudes, enhance empathy, and reduce aggression. All these aspects contribute to a more fulfilling and balanced life.

Gratitude's benefits extend beyond physical and mental health to every aspect of life.

In Conclusion

The science of gratitude is a burgeoning field, revealing the profound impact of this simple emotion on our lives. By fostering gratitude, we can enhance our physical health, improve our mental well-being, strengthen our relationships, and cultivate a more fulfilling life. All it takes is a moment to reflect on what we are thankful for daily.

As we progress in this book, we'll explore practical strategies for cultivating gratitude. But for now, let's take a moment to appreciate the power of gratitude - the ability to transform our health, minds, and lives in profound and measurable ways.

Interactive Activity: Gratitude Journaling

Objective: To help experience first-hand the benefits of practicing gratitude.

General Method Instructions:

1. Take a moment to sit comfortably and clear your mind.

2. Now, think about three things you are grateful for today. They can be big or small, from the taste of your morning coffee to a supportive friend.

3. Write these down in a notebook or digital document. Please describe why you're grateful for each and how they made you feel.

4. Repeat this activity every day for a week. At the end of the week, reflect on how you feel. Did you notice any changes in your mood, sleep, or overall well-being?

Alternative "Intentional" Method Instructions:

1. Take a moment to sit comfortably and clear your mind.

2. Now, think about one thing you are grateful for today. This can be big or small,

3. Write this down in a notebook or digital document if you feel inclined. This isn't always necessary. Describe why you're grateful for this one thing and how it made you feel.

4. Now go deeper into that one thing. Explore all aspects of all involved with this person, place, or thing. For example, if it's your comfy bed you're grateful for, think about everything

involved in getting that bed to you. From the farmers who grew the cotton or the technology of the synthetic fabric to all the people, equipment, processes and resources necessary to get the bed to your room.

5. Repeat this activity every day for a week. At the end of the week, reflect on how you feel. Did you notice any changes in your mood, sleep, or overall well-being?

Challenge: Gratitude Letter

Objective: To enhance readers' understanding of the social benefits of gratitude.

Instructions:

1. Think of someone who has significantly impacted your life but whom you've never properly thanked.

2. Write a letter expressing your appreciation for this person. Please explain why you're grateful and how they've positively influenced your life.

3. If you feel comfortable, share this letter with the person by mail, email, or in person.

Quiz: Understanding the Science of Gratitude

1. What neurotransmitter, often called the 'feel-good' neurotransmitter, is released when we express gratitude? a) Serotonin b) Dopamine c) Oxytocin d) Adrenaline

2. What hormone, known as the 'social bonding hormone,' is released when we experience positive social interactions, including expressing or receiving gratitude? a) Serotonin b) Dopamine c) Oxytocin d) Adrenaline

3. What are some of the psychological benefits of gratitude? a) Increased happiness b) Reduced depression c) Enhanced empathy d) All of the above

4. True or False: Practicing gratitude can improve sleep quality. a) True b) False

5. True or False: The habit of gratitude can change the brain's neural structures. a) True b) False

Answers: 1) b, 2) c, 3) d, 4) a, 5) a

References

1. Hill, P. L., Allemand, M., & Roberts, B. W. (2013). Examining the pathways between gratitude and self-rated physical health across adulthood. Personality and individual differences, 54(1), 92-96.

2. Wood, A. M., Joseph, S., & Maltby, J. (2008). Gratitude uniquely predicts satisfaction with life: Incremental validity above the domains and facets of the five-factor model. Personality and Individual Differences, 45(1), 49-54.

3. Emmons, R. A., & McCullough, M. E. (2003). Counting blessings versus burdens: an experimental investigation of gratitude and subjective well-being in daily life. Journal of personality and social psychology, 84(2), 377.

4. Tsang, J. A. (2006). Gratitude and prosocial behavior: An experimental test of gratitude. Cognition & Emotion, 20(1), 138-148.

5. Kashdan, T. B., Uswatte, G., & Julian, T. (2006). Gratitude and hedonic and eudaimonic well-being in Vietnam War veterans. Behavior research and therapy, 44(2), 177-199.

6. Kini, P., Wong, J., McInnis, S., Gabana, N., & Brown, J. W. (2016). The effects of gratitude expression on neural activity. NeuroImage, 128, 1-10.

7. Fox, G. R., Kaplan, J., Damasio, H., & Damasio, A. (2015). Neural correlates of gratitude. Frontiers in Psychology, 6, 1491.

8. Emmons, R. A., & Stern, R. (2013). Gratitude as a psychotherapeutic intervention. Journal of Clinical Psychology, 69(8), 846-855.

9. Jackowska, M., Brown, J., Ronaldson, A., & Steptoe, A. (2016). The impact of a brief gratitude intervention on subjective well-being, biology and sleep. Journal of Health Psychology, 21(10), 2207-2217.

10. Redwine, L. S., Henry, B. L., Pung, M. A., Wilson, K., Chinh, K., Knight, B., ... & Mills, P. J. (2016). Pilot randomized study of a gratitude journaling intervention on heart rate variability and inflammatory biomarkers in patients with stage B heart failure. Psychosomatic medicine, 78(6), 667.

11. Peterson, J. C., Charlson, M. E., Hoffman, Z., Wells, M. T., Wong, S. C., Hollenberg, J. P., ... & Allegrante, J. P. (2012). A randomized controlled trial of positive-affect induction to promote physical activity after percutaneous coronary intervention. Archives of Internal Medicine, 172(4), 329-336.

12. Segerstrom, S. C., & Sephton, S. E. (2010). Optimistic expectancies and cell-mediated immunity: The role of positive affect. Psychological science, 21(3), 448-455.

13. McCullough, M. E., Emmons, R. A., & Tsang, J. A. (2002). The grateful disposition: a conceptual and empirical topography. Journal of personality and social psychology, 82(1), 112.

14. Fredrickson, B. L., Tugade, M. M., Waugh, C. E., & Larkin, G. R. (2003). What good are positive emotions in crisis? A prospective study of resilience and emotions following the

terrorist attacks on the United States on September 11th, 2001. Journal of personality and social psychology, 84(2), 365.

15. Nelson, K. S., Layous, K., Cole, S. W., & Lyubomirsky, S. (2016). Do unto others or treat yourself? The effects of prosocial and self-focused behavior on psychological flourishing. Emotion, 16(6), 850.

16. Wood, A. M., Maltby, J., Gillett, R., Linley, P. A., & Joseph, S. (2008). The role of gratitude in the development of social support, stress, and depression: Two longitudinal studies. Journal of Research in Personality, 42(4), 854-871.

17. Ferris, D. L., Chen, M., & Lim, V. K. (2017). Comparing and contrasting workplace ostracism and incivility during a global pandemic. Journal of Applied Psychology, 102(12), 2078.

18. Chan, D. W. (2013). Subjective well-being of Hong Kong Chinese teachers: The contribution of gratitude, forgiveness, and the orientations to happiness. Teaching and Teacher Education, 32, 22-30.

19. Tennen, H., & Affleck, G. (2002). Benefit-finding and benefit-reminding. Handbook of positive psychology, 1, 584-597.

20. Fredrickson, B. L., Tugade, M. M., Waugh, C. E., & Larkin, G. R. (2003). What good are positive emotions in crisis? A prospective study of resilience and emotions following the terrorist attacks on the United States on September 11th, 2001. Journal of personality and social psychology, 84(2), 365.

Otto, K., Körner, A., & Steffens, G. M. (2015). Beliefs about benefits of adversity moderate the relationship between adverse life events and psychological health. Journal of Positive Psychology, 10(5), 446-458.

Lesson 3

Gratitude and Mindfulness

These two concepts of gratitude and mindfulness often appear together in the discourse of mental well-being and for a good reason. Gratitude and mindfulness intertwine and mutually reinforce each other. Let's unpack this relationship and explore how mindfulness enhances gratitude.

Relationship Between Mindfulness and Gratitude

The first question that may arise is: what precisely is the relationship between mindfulness and gratitude? To answer, let's first discuss what it means to practice being mindful, and briefly revisit the definition of gratitude.

Understanding Mindfulness

Mindfulness, a concept deeply rooted in Buddhist philosophy, refers to the practice of maintaining a moment-by-moment awareness of our thoughts, emotions, bodily sensations, and surrounding environment with openness and curiosity. It's about being fully engaged in the present moment without judgment, rather than being lost in thought or distracted by memories or future concerns. Like gratitude, research links mindfulness to a range of psychological and physiological benefits, including stress reduction, improved attention and memory, enhanced emotional well-being, and even a stronger immune system.

Gratitude is a positive emotional response that we perceive on giving or receiving a benefit from someone (either from another person or a higher power). It's about recognizing and appreciating the good things in life, both big and small.

The link between mindfulness and gratitude is the act of 'presence.' Mindfulness primes us to be present and fully engaged in the moment. By practicing mindfulness, we can enhance our capacity for gratitude. Mindfulness helps us slow down, pay attention, and appreciate the present moment, creating more opportunities for gratitude. Conversely, gratitude can deepen our practice of mindfulness. By fostering a positive mindset, gratitude can make it easier for us to stay present and engaged in the here and now. When we're present, we're more likely to notice and appreciate the good things happening around us, cultivating a natural sense of gratitude. Conversely, when we cultivate a sense of gratitude, we ground ourselves in the present moment, strengthening our mindfulness.

The Science Behind Gratitude and Mindfulness

Neuroscientific research has unveiled why gratitude and mindfulness are so beneficial. Both practices have been shown to activate areas of the brain associated with positive emotion, social connection, and attention. They can also reduce activity in areas linked to stress and negative emotions. On a physiological level, gratitude and mindfulness can lower blood pressure, reduce inflammation, and improve sleep, among other benefits.

The Benefits of Mindfulness in Enhancing Gratitude

Now, let's discuss how mindfulness can augment our gratitude practice. Mindfulness has several benefits that enhance gratitude:

1. **Increased Awareness:** Being mindful increases our awareness of the present moment. This heightened awareness allows us to notice and appreciate the small, everyday blessings in our lives, from a warm cup of coffee to a kind word from a friend, fostering a sense of gratitude.

2. **Overcoming Negativity Bias:** As humans, we are hard wired to pay more attention to negative experiences–a trait known as negativity bias. This bias can sometimes obscure our ability to recognize positive experiences. By consciously directing our attention and enabling us, mindfulness can help us combat this bias. By focusing on the positive, we foster a sense of gratitude.

3. **Improved Emotional Regulation:** Mindfulness enables us to better manage and respond to our emotions. This improved emotional regulation can help reduce reactive negative behaviors like anger or resentment, which often obstruct feelings of gratitude.

4. **Cultivating Patience:** The practice of mindfulness encourages patience—a quality that's also important in cultivating gratitude. By sitting with our experiences without rushing to judge or react, we learn to observe our lives more patiently. This patience can enhance our capacity to appreciate and be grateful for what we have.

Practical Ways to Cultivate Gratitude and Mindfulness

There are many practical ways to cultivate both gratitude and mindfulness. Techniques like keeping a gratitude journal, expressing thanks to others, and mindful meditation can be effective. Even simple acts, like savoring a meal or appreciating a beautiful sunset, can foster both gratitude and mindfulness. We'll discuss these in more detail later in the course.

The Impact of Gratitude and Mindfulness on Mental Health

Studies show that both gratitude and mindfulness have profound effects on mental health. They can ease symptoms of stress and anxiety, combat depression, and promote mental strength. They can also boost self-esteem and overall life satisfaction.

The Broader Benefits of Gratitude and Mindfulness

Beyond mental health, gratitude and mindfulness offer broader benefits. They can enhance personal relationships, improve productivity and job satisfaction, and foster resilience in the face of adversity. They also promote a sense of connectedness and community, contributing to a more compassionate and caring society.

Conclusion

The practices of gratitude and mindfulness offer a wealth of benefits, both individually and in synergy. By incorporating these practices into our daily lives, we can enhance our mental and physical well-being, nurture our relationships, and contribute to a more positive and compassionate society. The journey towards well-being is lifelong, and gratitude and mindfulness can be valuable companions along the way.

Interactive Activity:

Mindful Gratitude Exercise

For our interactive activity today, we'll engage in a simple yet powerful practice: a mindful gratitude exercise.

Find a quiet and comfortable space where you can sit without being disturbed for about 15 minutes. Close your eyes and take several deep breaths to center yourself in the present moment.

Let your mind wander through your day or week, observing each thought as it arises and falls away. As you do this, attempt to identify positive elements or experiences you feel grateful for. These could be significant events or small, everyday blessings.

Focus on these moments of gratitude, letting yourself feel the appreciation fully. After you've spent some time with these positive experiences, open your eyes and write them down in your gratitude journal.

Mindful Gratitude Practice

This is a simple activity that combines mindfulness and gratitude. Find a quiet space and take a few deep breaths to center yourself. Now, bring to mind something or someone you're grateful for. Spend a few moments reflecting on this. Notice the emotions that arise and any changes in your body. Allow yourself to fully feel the gratitude. Once you're done, write your experience in a journal.

Challenge: 7-Day Gratitude and Mindfulness Challenge

For the next seven days, commit to practicing mindfulness and expressing gratitude daily. Spend at least 10 minutes each day practicing mindfulness, focusing on your breath or your surroundings. Also, write three things you are grateful for each day. Try to do this mindfully and intentionally. Strive for authentic or even awe-inspiring gratitude. Notice any changes in your mood, stress level, or overall well-being at the end of the challenge.

You can also try taking a simpler approach: choose just one thing to appreciate, no matter how small. Then explore its deeper dimensions, discovering layers of gratitude within this single focus.

Consider your couch as an example. Start with its immediate comfort and softness. Then trace its journey: from the farmers growing cotton for its fabric, to the mill workers weaving the textiles, to the craftspeople assembling its frame. Picture the truck drivers transporting materials, the designers creating its form, and the store employees helping it reach your home. Your couch represents an intricate web of human effort and collaboration—all contributing to your daily comfort.

Quiz: Test Your Understanding of Gratitude and Mindfulness

1. What's gratitude? a. Feeling thankful for the positive aspects of life. b. A type of mindfulness practice. c. A way to reduce negative emotions. d. All of the above.

2. What's mindfulness? a. Being present in the moment without judgment. b. A type of meditation. c. A way to reduce stress. d. All of the above.

3. True or False: Gratitude and mindfulness can help improve mental health.

4. Which of the following is a way to cultivate gratitude and mindfulness? a. Keep a gratitude journal. b. Practice mindful meditation. c. Savor a meal or a beautiful view. d. All of the above.

5. True or False: Gratitude and mindfulness only have psychological benefits, not physical ones.

6. How does mindfulness enhance the practice of gratitude?

    a) It helps us dwell on past experiences.

    b) It promotes a focus on the negative aspects of our lives.

    c) It increases our awareness of the present moment, helping us recognize and appreciate positive experiences.

    d) It has no significant effect on gratitude.

7. What's the link between mindfulness and gratitude?

a) They are mutually exclusive practices with no common elements.

b) They both encourage ruminating on past experiences.

c) They both foster a focus on future ambitions.

d) They both enhance our presence and appreciation of the present moment.

Answers:

1. What's gratitude?

    • Answer: d. All of the above. Explanation: Gratitude is feeling thankful for the positive aspects of life, can be a type of mindfulness practice, and is a way to reduce negative emotions.

2. What's mindfulness?

    • Answer: d. All of the above. Explanation: Mindfulness is being present in the moment without judgment, is a type of meditation, and is a way to reduce stress.

3. True or False: Gratitude and mindfulness can help improve mental health.

    • Answer: True. Explanation: Studies show that gratitude and mindfulness both reduce symptoms of stress, anxiety, and depression, and improve overall well-being, thus positively affecting mental health.

4. Which of the following is a way to cultivate gratitude and mindfulness?

- Answer: d. All of the above. Explanation: Keeping a gratitude journal, practicing mindful meditation, and savoring a meal or a beautiful view are all ways to cultivate gratitude and mindfulness.

5. True or False: Gratitude and mindfulness only have psychological benefits, not physical ones.

  - Answer: False. Explanation: Studies have shown that both gratitude and mindfulness offer physical benefits, such as improved sleep, lower blood pressure, and a stronger immune system, besides their psychological benefits.

6. c

7. d

By understanding and practicing mindfulness, you've added a valuable tool to your gratitude toolkit. In our next lesson, we'll examine various techniques for incorporating gratitude into your daily life. Until then, enjoy your journey of mindful gratitude.

References:

1. Emmons, R. A., & McCullough, M. E. (2003). Counting blessings versus burdens: An experimental investigation of gratitude and subjective well-being in daily life. Journal of Personality and Social Psychology, 84(2), 377.

2. Kabat-Zinn, J. (2003). Mindfulness-based interventions in context: Past, present, and future. Clinical Psychology: Science and Practice, 10(2), 144-156.

3. Wood, A. M., Froh, J. J., & Geraghty, A. W. (2010). Gratitude and well-being: A review and theoretical integration. Clinical Psychology Review, 30(7), 890-905.

4. Brown, K. W., & Ryan, R. M. (2003). The benefits of being present: Mindfulness and its role in psychological well-being. Journal of Personality and Social Psychology, 84(4), 822.

5. Algoe, S. B. (2012). Find, remind, and bind: The functions of gratitude in everyday relationships. Social and Personality Psychology Compass, 6(6), 455-469.

Lesson 4

The Impact of Gratitude on Relationships

In this lesson, we'll explore an exciting and crucial aspect of gratitude: its influence on relationships. In this chapter, we'll uncover how gratitude can enhance our relationships, backed by empirical evidence. We'll provide strategies to cultivate this vital emotion within our interpersonal connections later in the lessons, specifically focusing on gratitude practices. For this lesson, we'll concentrate on the evidence and the possible mechanisms of the beneficial effects of gratitude on relationships.

Gratitude isn't merely a personal emotion; it's inherently social and plays a crucial role in our relationships. We often feel gratitude in response to others' actions - when they do something kind or helpful, particularly when it's not obligatory (Algoe, 2012). Gratitude can act as a social glue that binds people together, strengthens existing relationships, and fosters new ones. It encourages mutual care and understanding, fosters connection, and helps individuals navigate the social world (Algoe, 2012).

Relationships of all types, whether they're with family, friends, romantic partners, or colleagues, are fundamental to our well-being and happiness. They provide us with support, care, companionship, and love. As such, understanding the role gratitude plays in our relationships can be transformative, not only for our social connections, but also for our overall well-being.

Gratitude: Strengthening Bonds and Deepening Connections

Gratitude's effects on relationships are well-documented in scientific literature. Many studies have explored the role of gratitude in relationships, underscoring its power to improve relationship satisfaction, deepen emotional connections, and foster long-lasting bonds.

- **Family Relationships:**

  - In family relationships, gratitude can act as a social glue, fostering connectivity and mutual appreciation. A study by Gordon et al. (2012) found that gratitude played a significant role in marital satisfaction, with couples who expressed gratitude to each other reporting stronger relationships.

  - Froh et al. (2010) found that children and adolescents who expressed gratitude showed increased positive attitudes and behaviors towards their families. This suggests that gratitude can be influential in shaping family dynamics, promoting cohesion and harmony.

- **Friendships and Acquaintances:**

  - In the sphere of friendships, studies have shown that gratitude can deepen bonds and increase closeness. For example, Algoe et al. (2013) found that expressions of gratitude served as a relationship strengthener among friends. Expressing gratitude made recipients more likely to perceive the relationship as meaningful and supportive.

- Demonstrating gratitude can make us more likable and foster new friendships. For instance, a study by Williams and Bartlett (2015) found that expressing gratitude to a new acquaintance can make them more likely to seek an ongoing relationship.

- **Romantic Relationships**

  - Practicing gratitude enhances romantic relationships. According to a study by Algoe et al. (2012), expressing gratitude to one's partner not only increases feelings of relationship satisfaction and connection, but also predicts future relationship quality and longevity.

  - Gordon et al. (2012) found that gratitude in romantic relationships can predict marital satisfaction, helping couples feel more connected and satisfied. Partners who express gratitude can boost their relationship satisfaction and deepen their bond.

- **Work Relationships**

  - In the workplace, gratitude can foster a positive work environment and improve employee morale. A study by Grant and Gino (2010) reported that when leaders expressed gratitude for their employees' hard work, employees felt more motivated and reported higher levels of job satisfaction. Their study revealed that expressing gratitude can boost individuals' sense of self-worth and motivate them to be more productive. This suggests that gratitude can contribute to a more positive and productive work environment.

The Underlying Mechanisms

Understanding why gratitude has such a profound impact on our relationships involves delving deeper into the psychological and neurobiological mechanisms at play. Here are some of the key theories and findings from the field:

- **Emotional Reinforcement:** Gratitude can serve as a powerful emotional reinforcement within relationships. When someone expresses gratitude to us, it's a positive affirmation of our actions and intentions. This positive reinforcement can make us more likely to repeat these behaviors, helping to solidify positive interaction patterns within our relationships.

- **Increased Prosocial Behavior:** Research has shown that gratitude can lead to increased prosocial behavior—that is, actions intended to benefit others. Acts of kindness or generosity often trigger feelings of gratitude, and these feelings can motivate us to pay it forward. This can create a positive feedback loop of kindness and appreciation within our relationships, further strengthening our bonds.

- **Boosting Perceived Reciprocity:** Expressing gratitude can increase perceived reciprocity in relationships, making us feel more balanced in our give-and-take dynamics. This sense of reciprocity is an essential component of healthy relationships, fostering feelings of fairness and mutual respect.

- **Neurobiological Effects:** Neurobiologically, gratitude activates regions of the brain associated with social bonding, stress relief, and pleasure (such as the hypothalamus and the ventral tegmental area). Over time, regular expressions of gratitude can lead to long-term changes in these neural circuits, promoting sustained feelings of closeness and satisfaction in our relationships.

- **The 'Find-Remind-and-Bind' Theory:** This theory proposed by Algoe (2012) explains how gratitude influences relationships:

  - **Find:** Gratitude helps us identify and 'find' people who care for us and show us kindness.

  - **Remind:** Gratitude serves to 'remind' us of the existing supportive relationships in our lives.

  - **Bind:** Gratitude helps to 'bind' us closer to these people, fostering stronger and more meaningful connections.

This theory underscores the reciprocal nature of gratitude in relationships: when one person expresses gratitude, it often leads to a positive feedback loop where both individuals feel more appreciated and satisfied with the relationship.

- **Enhancing Self-Worth:** Gratitude can also enhance our sense of self-worth. When someone expresses gratitude to us, it validates our actions and reinforces the belief that we are valued and appreciated. This boost to self-worth can lead to increased confidence and satisfaction in our relationships.

- **Promoting Positive Communication:** Gratitude promotes positive communication. By focusing on what we appreciate about others and expressing it, we are more likely to communicate in a positive, affirming way. This can foster better conflict resolution, increased understanding, and more constructive discussions.

A range of psychological and neurobiological mechanisms work together to foster mutual appreciation underpinned the impact of gratitude on relationships, increase prosocial behavior, enhance communication, and strengthens emotional bonds. Each expression of gratitude sets off a chain reaction of positivity that can enhance the quality and depth of our relationships.

The Transformative Power of Gratitude

The significance of gratitude in relationships can't be overstated. Gratitude holds transformative power to deepen our bonds, improve mutual understanding, and foster a more empathetic society. Gratitude has the potential to transform our relationships, making them stronger, more resilient, and more fulfilling. With a greater understanding of gratitude's powerful impact on our relationships, we can consciously incorporate it into our interactions. Whether with a romantic partner, friends, family, or colleagues, practicing gratitude can significantly enhance the quality of our relationships, fostering deeper connections and shared joy. Remember, cultivating gratitude isn't just about improving our individual lives, but also about enhancing our relationships and the communities we belong to.

Remember that, like any skill, the ability to express and feel gratitude in relationships requires consistent practice. So, let's embark on this journey, allowing gratitude to enrich our social lives.

Until then, keep noticing, appreciating, and expressing your gratitude. Because every thank you, every sign, acknowledgement, and expression of appreciation matters.

Interactive Activity: Gratitude Letter

For this activity, you're going to write a gratitude letter. This is a letter you write to someone who has made a significant positive impact on your life, but whom you've never properly thanked. Spend 20-30 minutes writing this letter. Be specific about what they did, why you're grateful, and how their actions affected your life.

While you don't have to send the letter, often people choose to, and it can be a powerful experience to share your feelings of gratitude with the person who inspired them.

Challenge: Gratitude Expression Week

For one week, make it a goal to express your gratitude daily to the people in your life. This could be a spouse, a friend, a colleague, or even a helpful stranger. It doesn't have to be for anything grand; simple, everyday acts of kindness can be just as meaningful.

The key is to be genuine and specific in your expression of gratitude. Instead of just saying "Thank you," explain why you're thankful and what it meant to you.

At the end of the week, reflect on how this challenge affected your feelings and your relationships. Did you notice any changes in your interactions or emotional state?

Quiz: Understanding the Impact of Gratitude on Relationships

1. Which of the following is NOT a benefit of expressing gratitude in relationships? a) Increased relationship satisfaction b) Enhanced communication c) Reduced empathy d) Strengthened emotional bonds

2. The 'find-remind-and-bind' theory is associated with: a) Negative emotions b) Gratitude c) Anger management d) Stress reduction

3. Gratitude can reduce negative emotions and pave the way for: a) Increased resentment b) More conflict c) More positive emotions d) None of the above

4. According to research, expressing gratitude can increase perceived reciprocity in relationships. True or False?

5. In neurobiology, gratitude activates regions of the brain associated with: a) Fear and anger b) Social bonding and pleasure c) Hunger and thirst d) None of the above

(Answers: 1c, 2b, 3c, 4True, 5b)

References

- Algoe, S. B. (2012). Find, remind, and bind: The functions of gratitude in everyday relationships. Social and Personality Psychology Compass, 6(6), 455-469.

- Algoe, S. B., Gable, S. L., & Maisel, N. C. (2013). It's the little things: Everyday gratitude as a booster shot for romantic relationships. Personal Relationships, 20(2), 217-233.

- Algoe, S. B., Haidt, J., & Gable, S. L. (2008). Beyond reciprocity: Gratitude and relationships in everyday life. Emotion, 8(3), 425.

- Froh, J. J., Yurkewicz, C., & Kashdan, T. B. (2009). Gratitude and subjective well-being in early adolescence: Examining gender differences. Journal of adolescence, 32(3), 633-650.

- Gordon, A. M., Impett, E. A., Kogan, A., Oveis, C., & Keltner, D. (2012). To have and to hold: Gratitude promotes relationship maintenance in intimate bonds. Journal of Personality and Social Psychology, 103(2), 257.

- Grant, A. M., & Gino, F. (2010). A little thanks goes a long way: Explaining why gratitude expressions motivate prosocial behavior. Journal of Personality and Social Psychology, 98(6), 946.

- Williams, L. A., & Bartlett, M. Y. (2015). Warm thanks: Gratitude expression facilitates social affiliation in new relationships via perceived warmth. Emotion, 15(1), 1-5.

Lesson 5

The Impact of Gratitude on Positive Emotions

This lesson focuses on an essential aspect of gratitude: its relationship with positive emotions, such as joy, peace, and happiness.

Emotions profoundly shape our lives, affecting our thoughts, decisions, and overall well-being. Positive emotions can enhance our resilience, creativity, and even our physical health. As we delve into the research on gratitude and positive emotions, you'll discover how cultivating an attitude of gratitude can lead to an increase in these beneficial emotional states.

Gratitude and Positive Emotions: An Inextricable Link

Gratitude doesn't just make us feel good in the moment. It also helps cultivate a broad range of positive emotions, serving as a catalyst for happiness, joy, peace, and more. Here's what science has to say:

Gratitude and Happiness

The link between gratitude and happiness is well-established. A study by Emmons and McCullough (2003) found that individuals who kept a gratitude journal reported significantly higher levels of happiness compared to those who didn't. This suggests that the regular practice of gratitude can lead to sustained increases in happiness.

Gratitude and Joy

Gratitude can also enhance feelings of joy. When we appreciate the good in our lives, we experience a sense of pleasure and satisfaction, leading to feelings of joy. For example, a study by Watkins et al. (2003) demonstrated that gratitude exercises led to increased joy among participants.

Gratitude and Peace

Gratitude can contribute to feelings of peace by shifting our focus from what's wrong in our lives to what's right. By appreciating what we have, we can reduce feelings of lack or dissatisfaction, leading to a greater sense of peace. A study by Wood et al. (2009) revealed that gratitude was associated with lower levels of stress and depression, suggesting that it may foster a sense of peace and well-being.

Satisfaction

Gratitude can also contribute to feelings of satisfaction. When we appreciate what we have, instead of focusing on what we lack, it can lead to a greater sense of contentment and satisfaction with our lives. Research has found that individuals who practice gratitude report higher levels of life satisfaction.

Optimism

Studies have also linked gratitude to optimism. By focusing on the positive aspects of our lives and appreciating them, we can cultivate a more optimistic outlook. Studies have shown that people who regularly practice gratitude have a more positive future-oriented perspective.

Hope

Gratitude can foster hope by helping us appreciate the positive aspects of our current situation, which can make us more hopeful about the future. In challenging times, gratitude can help us focus on our strengths and resources, fostering a sense of hope and positivity.

Compassion

Gratitude can also boost feelings of compassion. Recognizing the kindness of others can foster empathy and compassion, as we're more likely to reciprocate these positive actions. Research shows that gratitude practices can increase our empathetic responses and willingness to help others.

The Underlying Mechanisms

So, how does gratitude cultivate these positive emotions? Let's explore some of the key mechanisms:

- **Shifting Attention to the Positive:** Gratitude can shift our attention away from negative aspects of our lives towards the positive. This reframing can help us recognize and appreciate the good, leading to an increase in positive emotions.

- **Savoring Positive Experiences:** Gratitude helps us savor our positive experiences. By appreciating these moments, we can prolong the positive emotions associated with them, which can enhance our overall well-being and happiness.

- **Reducing Negative Emotions:** Gratitude can reduce negative emotions like anger, envy, and regret. By focusing on what we're grateful for, we are less likely to dwell on negative experiences or emotions, paving the way for more joy, peace, and happiness.

- **Promoting Coping and Resilience:** Gratitude serves as a powerful lens for navigating stress and adversity. By helping us view challenges within a broader context, it fosters resilience and reveals opportunities for growth, even in our most difficult moments.

Gratitude has a profound impact on our emotional well-being. By cultivating gratitude, we can boost our happiness, increase joy, foster a sense of hope and peace, boost feelings of compassion, and enrich optimism. The beauty of gratitude is that it's accessible to us all. Every moment provides an opportunity to notice, appreciate, and express gratitude, enhancing positive emotions and overall well-being.

Until our next lesson, keep expressing gratitude and reaping its emotional rewards.

Interactive Activity: Gratitude Journaling

Start a gratitude journal. Each day for a week, write three things you're grateful for. They can be big or small, significant or trivial, but the key is to reflect deeply on what these things mean to you and why they bring you joy, peace, or happiness.

At the end of the week, take some time to reflect on your entries and notice any patterns or recurring themes.

If finding three things to be grateful for each day feels more like a task or assignment, try finding one thing to be grateful for as we did in the exercise in lesson 3, the "7-Day Gratitude and Mindfulness Challenge".

Challenge: Daily Gratitude Share

For one week, besides your gratitude journal, share something you're grateful for each day with someone else. This could be in person, through a phone call, or via a text message or email. This challenge expresses your gratitude out loud, which can amplify its positive effects. Also, your shared gratitude might inspire positivity in the person you share it with.

Quiz: Understanding the Impact of Gratitude on Positive Emotions

1. Studies have shown gratitude increases which of the following emotions? a) Happiness b) Joy c) Peace d) All of the above

2. Gratitude can shift our attention from: a) Positive aspects of our lives to negative ones b) Negative aspects of our lives to positive ones c) Neither a nor b d) Both a and b

3. Which of the following is NOT a way that gratitude can enhance positive emotions? a) By promoting coping and resilience b) By increasing negative emotions c) By helping us savor positive experiences d) By shifting our attention to the positive

4. Researchers have shown that writing a gratitude letter increases feelings of: a) Anger b) Resentment c) Love d) None of the above

5. According to research, expressing gratitude can increase life satisfaction. True or False?

(Answers: 1d, 2b, 3b, 3c, 4c, 5True)

References

- Emmons, R. A., & McCullough, M. E. (2003). Counting blessings versus burdens: An experimental investigation of gratitude and subjective well-being in daily life. Journal of Personality and Social Psychology, 84(2), 377.

- Watkins, P. C., Woodward, K., Stone, T., & Kolts, R. L. (2003). Gratitude and happiness: Development of a measure of gratitude, and relationships with subjective well-being. Social Behavior and Personality: An International Journal, 31(5), 431-451.

- Wood, A. M., Joseph, S., & Maltby, J. (2009). Gratitude predicts psychological well-being above the Big Five facets. Personality and Individual Differences, 46(4), 443-447.

- Algoe, S. B., Haidt, J., & Gable, S. L. (2008). Beyond reciprocity: Gratitude and relationships in everyday life. Emotion, 8(3), 425.

- Emmons, R. A., & McCullough, M. E. (2003). Counting blessings versus burdens: An experimental investigation of gratitude and subjective well-being in daily life. Journal of Personality and Social Psychology, 84(2), 377.

- Wood, A. M., Maltby, J., Gillett, R., Linley, P. A., & Joseph, S. (2008). The role of gratitude in the development of social support, stress, and depression: Two longitudinal studies. Journal of Research in Personality, 42(4), 854-871.

- Snyder, C. R., Ilardi, S. S., Michael, S. T., & Cheavens, J. (2000). Hope theory: Updating a common process for psychological change. In C. R. Snyder & R. E. Ingram (Eds.), Handbook of psychological change: Psychotherapy processes & practices for the 21st century (p. 128–153). John Wiley & Sons.

- Bartlett, M. Y., & DeSteno, D. (2006). Gratitude and prosocial behavior: Helping when it costs you. Psychological Science, 17(4), 319-325.

Lesson 6

The Impact of Gratitude on Life Satisfaction

In this lesson, we'll explore a crucial facet of gratitude: its profound impact on life satisfaction.

Gratitude is more than just a momentary feeling; it's a mindset that can alter our perspective on life. Scientific literature consistently shows a positive relationship between gratitude and life satisfaction. Life satisfaction, a key aspect of subjective well-being, refers to the overall assessment of the quality and fulfillment of our lives. As we navigate through life's difficulties, fostering a sense of satisfaction and fulfillment is paramount. As you'll discover in this lesson, gratitude can significantly enhance our feelings of life satisfaction, offering a more contented and fulfilling life.

Gratitude: Enhancing Life Satisfaction

A landmark study by Emmons and McCullough (2003) found that individuals who kept a gratitude journal reported higher levels of life satisfaction compared to those who didn't. This suggests that cultivating an attitude of gratitude can contribute to a more satisfying life.

In another study, Wood, Joseph, and Maltby (2008) found that gratitude could predict life satisfaction above and beyond the effect of personality traits. This highlights the unique role of gratitude in promoting life satisfaction.

A study by Watkins et al. (2003) showed that gratitude was related to a 10% improvement in life satisfaction, suggesting that gratitude can have a substantial impact on how we perceive and experience our lives. Other benefits of gratitude on life satisfaction include:

- **Fostering Positive Life Appraisal:** Gratitude fosters a positive appraisal of our life circumstances. By focusing on the positive aspects of our lives and expressing appreciation for them, we can enhance our overall evaluation of our life quality. In doing so, we cultivate a more optimistic and contented outlook, which is central to life satisfaction.

- **Studies show that gratitude reduces materialistic goals and attitudes.** By practicing appreciation for what we already have, we can reduce the desire for more material possessions, thus promoting contentment and satisfaction with our current circumstances.

- **Cultivating Optimism:** Gratitude cultivates optimism about the future. By appreciating the positive aspects of our present, we can maintain a more hopeful and positive outlook on our future. This optimistic perspective can enhance our overall life satisfaction.

- **Enhancing Self-Esteem:** Gratitude can enhance self-esteem, a crucial component of life satisfaction. When we appreciate our accomplishments and virtues, we can boost our self-esteem. Recognizing the role of others in our successes can foster a sense of interconnectedness and mutual respect, subsequently enhancing our life satisfaction.

- **Facilitating Coping and Stress Management:** Gratitude can facilitate better coping and stress management, contributing to greater life satisfaction. By appreciating the positive aspects of challenging situations, we can manage stress more effectively. Gratitude promotes resilience, helping us navigate through adversity and emerge stronger.

- **Encouraging Forgiveness:** Gratitude encourages forgiveness, which can enhance life satisfaction. By focusing on the positive aspects of our relationships and expressing gratitude for them, we can develop a more forgiving attitude. This can help us let go of resentment and bitterness, leading to healthier relationships and greater life satisfaction.

- **Promoting Physical Health:** Gratitude can even have physical health benefits, such as improved sleep and reduced symptoms of illness, which can indirectly enhance life satisfaction. Healthier individuals are more capable of enjoying and taking part fully in their lives, contributing to an overall higher sense of life satisfaction.

In summary, gratitude fosters life satisfaction through multiple pathways, from enhancing our appraisal of life, reducing materialism, fostering optimism, and promoting forgiveness, to improving our physical health. By cultivating an attitude of gratitude, we can enhance our life satisfaction and overall well-being.

Underlying Mechanisms: How Does Gratitude Enhance Life Satisfaction?

Now that we've looked at the evidence, let's try to understand why and how gratitude works to enhance life satisfaction.

- **Positive Reframing:** Gratitude encourages a positive reframing of our experiences. Instead of focusing on what's wrong or lacking in our lives, gratitude helps us appreciate what's good and abundant. This shift in perspective can enhance life satisfaction by promoting a more positive and appreciative view of our life circumstances.

- **Boosting Positive Emotions:** Gratitude can boost positive emotions, which are closely linked to life satisfaction. When we appreciate the good in our lives, we often experience a surge of positive emotions, like joy, happiness, and love. Over time, these enhanced positive emotions can contribute to greater life satisfaction.

- **Enhancing Resilience:** Gratitude can enhance our resilience, helping us to navigate challenges and adversity more effectively. It allows us to view difficulties in a broader context and recognize the potential for growth and learning in challenging situations. This increased resilience can lead to greater life satisfaction.

- **Promoting Healthy Relationships:** Gratitude can promote healthier and more satisfying relationships. As we've learned in a previous lesson, gratitude can strengthen bonds, improve communication, and enhance mutual appreciation in relationships. Given the central role of relationships in our lives, these improvements can significantly contribute to life satisfaction.

In conclusion, gratitude is a powerful tool for enhancing life satisfaction. It helps us appreciate the good in our lives, boosts positive emotions, enhances resilience, and promotes healthier relationships. By cultivating an attitude of gratitude, we can lead a more fulfilling and satisfying life.

Until our next lesson, keep recognizing, appreciating, and expressing gratitude, because every moment of gratitude adds to a more satisfying life.

Interactive Activity: Gratitude Collage

Create a Gratitude Collage. Collect pictures, quotes, and mementos of things you're grateful for and assemble them into a collage. This can be a physical collage on poster board or a digital one using a program like PowerPoint or Canva. The goal is to create a visual representation of all the things that bring you joy, peace, and satisfaction in your life.

Challenge: Daily Gratitude Reflection

For the next week, spend a few moments each day reflecting on something you're grateful for. This could be an event, a person, an accomplishment, or something as simple as a beautiful sunset. Reflect on why you're grateful for it and how it contributes to your overall life satisfaction. At the end of the week, reflect on the impact this exercise has had on your sense of life satisfaction.

Quiz: Understanding the Impact of Gratitude on Life Satisfaction

1. According to research, gratitude can foster life satisfaction by:
    a) Increasing negative emotions b) Reducing positive emotions
    c) Fostering positive life appraisal d) Encouraging materialistic
    attitudes

2. Which of the following is NOT a way that gratitude can
    enhance life satisfaction? a) By promoting forgiveness b) By
    enhancing self-esteem c) By reducing resilience d) By fostering
    positive life appraisal.

3. True or False: Gratitude can improve physical health, which
    can indirectly enhance life satisfaction.

4. According to studies, which of the following can be enhanced
    by gratitude, contributing to life satisfaction? a) Optimism b)
    Self-esteem c) Coping and stress management d) All of the
    above

5. The act of expressing gratitude can lead to a more _____
    outlook on our future. a) Pessimistic b) Optimistic c) Neutral
    d) None of the above

(Answers: 1c, 2c, 3True, 4d, 5b)

References

- Emmons, R. A., & McCullough, M. E. (2003). Counting blessings versus burdens: An experimental investigation of gratitude and subjective well-being in daily life. Journal of Personality and Social Psychology, 84(2), 377.

- Watkins, P. C., Woodward, K., Stone, T., & Kolts, R. L. (2003). Gratitude and happiness: Development of a measure of gratitude, and relationships with subjective well-being. Social Behavior and Personality: an international journal, 31(5), 431-451.

- Wood, A. M., Joseph, S., & Maltby, J. (2009). Gratitude predicts psychological well-being above the Big Five facets. Personality and Individual Differences, 46(4), 443-447.

- Polak, E. L., & McCullough, M. E. (2006). Is gratitude an alternative to materialism? Journal of Happiness Studies, 7(3), 343-360.

- Wood, A. M., Maltby, J., Gillett, R., Linley, P. A., & Joseph, S. (2008). The role of gratitude in the development of social support, stress, and depression: Two longitudinal studies. Journal of Research in Personality, 42(4), 854-871.

- Kong, F., Ding, K., & Zhao, J. (2015). The relationships among gratitude, self-esteem, social support and life satisfaction among undergraduate students. Journal of Happiness Studies, 16(2), 477-489.

- Wood, A. M., Joseph, S., & Linley, P. A. (2007). Coping style as a psychological resource of grateful people. Journal of Social and Clinical Psychology, 26(9), 1076-1093.

- Toussaint, L., & Friedman, P. (2009). Forgiveness, gratitude, and well-being: The mediating role of affect and beliefs. Journal of Happiness Studies, 10(6), 635-654.

- Jackowska, M., Brown, J., Ronaldson, A., & Steptoe, A. (2016). The impact of a brief gratitude intervention on subjective well-being, biology and sleep. Journal of Health Psychology, 21(10), 2207-2217.

Practical Strategies for Cultivating Gratitude

In this lesson, we'll dive into practical strategies for cultivating gratitude in our daily lives. We find the beauty of gratitude not only in its potential benefits but also in how it can be integrated into our daily routines, responses, and mindset. Let's explore some of these strategies:

The Gratitude Journal

One of the most effective and widely researched strategies is keeping a gratitude journal. Jotting down a few things you're grateful for each day can have significant beneficial effects.

- **Understanding Gratitude Journaling** - Gratitude Journaling, at its core, involves regularly jotting down things for which you're grateful. This could be anything from a delicious meal, a kind gesture from a stranger, a beautiful sunset, or a personal achievement. By actively seeking and documenting these positive aspects of our lives, we're training our brains to notice and focus on the positive, rather than dwelling on the negatives (Emmons & McCullough, 2003).

  The beauty of gratitude journaling lies in its flexibility. You can adapt the practice to your preferences—journal daily or weekly, write in the morning or at night, list simple bullet points or write detailed entries—the choice is yours. The key is consistency and genuine reflection on the experiences that bring you gratitude (Seligman, Steen, Park, & Peterson, 2005).

- **The Science Behind Gratitude Journaling** Gratitude Journaling isn't just a feel-good practice—it's backed by a growing body of research in the field of positive psychology. Studies have found that those who maintain a gratitude journal experience a host of benefits, from improved mood and reduced stress to better physical health (Emmons & McCullough, 2003).

  - **Mental Health:** A study by Emmons and McCullough (2003) uncovered that participants who wrote about things they were grateful for were more optimistic and felt better about their lives compared to those who focused on hassles or neutral events.

  - **Physical Health:** Interestingly, the same study also revealed that those who kept a gratitude journal reported fewer physical symptoms and were more likely to exercise regularly. Gratitude, it seems, not only affects our minds but also our bodies.

  - **Sleep:** A study by Wood, Joseph, Lloyd, and Atkins (2009) demonstrated that individuals who kept a gratitude journal reported improved sleep quality. This could be because focusing on positive events before bed may help reduce worry and negativity, which often interfere with sleep.

  - **Relationships:** According to a study by Lambert, Fincham, and Stillman (2012), expressing gratitude to a partner can improve the quality of the relationship, making both partners feel more positive toward each other and more comfortable expressing relationship concerns.

- **How to Start a Gratitude Journal:** Starting a gratitude journal is straightforward, but there are some tips that can enhance the effectiveness of this practice:

  - **Choose a Journal:** Find a journal that suits your style—be it a fancy leather-bound notebook, a simple notepad, or a digital journaling app.

  - **Set a Routine:** Decide when and how often you'll write. Many find it helpful to journal at the start or end of the day.

  - **List the Good:** Write things for which you're grateful. Aim for at least three, but list more if you like!

  - **Details Matter:** Instead of writing superficial lists, dive into the details of each item. Describe why it made you feel grateful.

  - **Negative into Positive:** Challenge yourself to find the silver lining in difficult situations. This is critically important and most of us resist this. The reason for this is our individual perspective. We believe the situation dictates that perspective, that we don't have the option to choose our perspective. However, we have a choice. It may not feel true because our choice of perspective appears to be instantaneous, but it's not. This is because our choice of perspective is habitual. That habit chooses a negative perspective or what I have termed as the "victim path" or victim perspective. We'll discuss this in more depth outside of this course.

- **Review Regularly:** Take time to review past entries. This can serve as a powerful reminder of the positives in your life, especially during challenging times.

- **The Subtleties of Gratitude Journaling**

  - While it might seem simple on the surface, effective gratitude journaling requires mindfulness, sincerity, and a dash of creativity. It's not enough to simply list things you're thankful for—you should engage with the practice, exploring how each item affects your life and emotions.

  - For instance, instead of writing, "I'm grateful for my friend," you might delve deeper: "I'm grateful for my friend, Anna, who always listens to me without judgment. Her open-mindedness makes me feel valued and understood." This way, you not only identify a source of gratitude, but also explore why it's significant to you.

- **Overcoming Barriers to Gratitude Journaling** - Like any habit, gratitude journaling can sometimes feel challenging to maintain. You might find it repetitive or struggle to come up with new entries. Here are a few strategies to overcome common barriers:

  - **Repetition:** If your entries felt repetitive, look for unique, small moments of joy or kindness in your day. Alternatively, inspect the same sources of gratitude—how does gratitude develop or manifest in different ways?

  - **Writer's Block:** Some days, you might struggle to identify things you're grateful for. If this happens, try to shift your perspective. For instance, even challenging situations can have silver linings.

- Lack of Time: If finding time to journal is a challenge, consider integrating it into an existing routine, like during breakfast or before bedtime.

- Sustaining Your Gratitude Journaling Practice

- The key to sustaining gratitude journaling (or any habit) is to make it enjoyable and meaningful. Here are some tips:

- Personalization: Personalize your journal to make it an object you cherish. This might mean using a beautiful notebook, a favorite pen, or a digital platform you enjoy.

- Incorporation: Incorporate the journaling into a routine you already have. This can help ensure it doesn't feel like an additional task, but a natural part of your day.

- Flexibility: Be flexible. If you miss a day, simply resume the next. If daily journaling is too much, try every other day or even once a week.

- **Further Study: Beyond Self-Improvement** - While the benefits of gratitude journaling for self-improvement are well-documented, it's also worth considering how the practice can improve our relationships and contribute to a more empathetic society. By regularly practicing gratitude, we cultivate a mindset that recognizes and appreciates the positive in others. This can lead to more compassionate interactions, reinforcing social bonds and fostering a sense of community (Algoe, 2012).

Gratitude Letters or Visits

Writing a letter of gratitude to someone who has positively affected your life, and if possible, delivering it in person, can be a powerful practice. Research by Seligman, Steen, Park, and Peterson (2005) found that participants who wrote and delivered a letter of gratitude reported significant increases in happiness and decreases in depressive symptoms.

Gratitude Reminders

Setting up gratitude reminders can be an effective way to make gratitude a daily habit. This could be an alarm on your phone or a note on your mirror reminding you to reflect on what you're grateful for. Over time, this can help to shift your focus towards the positive aspects of your life.

Mindful Gratitude Meditations

Mindfulness meditation can be a powerful tool for cultivating gratitude. By focusing your attention on the present moment and acknowledging the positive aspects of your experience, you can foster a deeper sense of appreciation and gratitude. Kabat-Zinn's (1994) mindfulness-based stress reduction program includes gratitude as a key component.

Gratitude Prompts

Using gratitude prompts can be a useful strategy, especially if you find it challenging to come up with things you're grateful for. Prompts can be questions or statements designed to guide your reflection, such as "What's something that made you smile today?" or "Think about someone who did something nice for you recently."

Expressing Gratitude to Others

Regularly expressing gratitude to others, either verbally or in writing, can help to strengthen your relationships and enhance your own feelings of gratitude. Studies, such as Algoe, Gable, and Maisel (2010), show that gratitude expressions can lead to improved relationship quality and mutual feelings of connection and satisfaction.

Gratitude in Challenging Times

Even in challenging times, there are opportunities for gratitude. By focusing on what you can learn from a difficult situation or how it may lead to growth, you can cultivate gratitude, even in adversity.

The "Three Good Things" Practice

At the end of each day, reflect on three good things that happened. They don't have to be major events; even small moments of joy or success count. This practice, as per Seligman et al. (2005), can significantly increase happiness and reduce depressive symptoms.

There are many ways to cultivate an attitude of gratitude, and different strategies may suit different individuals. The key is consistency. By regularly practicing gratitude, we can reap its many benefits, from enhanced well-being to improved relationships and greater life satisfaction. Remember, practicing gratitude is flexible and adaptable—what matters is that you commit to it and make it a regular part of your life.

Through this lesson, we have covered the ins and outs of gratitude journaling as well as other gratitude practice techniques. We looked at the foundation of these practices, the scientific backing, implementation strategies, barriers, and potential for long-term sustainability and broader societal impact. As you venture into this practice, remember that patience and consistency are key. Enjoy the journey and reap the benefits of a grateful heart.

Interactive Activity: Starting Your Gratitude Journal

Now, it's your turn! Begin your gratitude journal by following the steps outlined above. Commit to writing in it for the next week. Remember, there's no right or wrong way to do this—what's most important is that it feels meaningful to you.

Bonus Activity: Create a Gratitude Jar. Find a jar and some small pieces of paper. Each day, write one thing you're grateful for and put it in the jar. This can be something big or small, from a person you appreciate to a pleasant moment in your day. At the end of the week, read through all the notes to remind yourself of the good in your life.

Challenge: The "Three Good Things" Challenge

For one week, practice the "Three Good Things" exercise each night before bed. Write three good things that happened to you during the day and why they were good. They don't need to be significant events; even simple, everyday things count. Reflect on how this practice affects your mood and perspective.

Quiz: Understanding Practical Strategies for Cultivating Gratitude

1. Which of the following is a well-researched strategy for cultivating gratitude? a) Daily gratitude journaling b) Writing gratitude letters c) Mindful gratitude meditations d) All the above.

2. True or False: The practice of gratitude is only beneficial during positive life events and circumstances.

3. The "Three Good Things" practice involves: a) Thinking of three things you're grateful for each week b) Reflecting on three good things that happened each day c) Writing a letter of gratitude to three people d) None of the above

4. Setting up gratitude reminders can: a) Make gratitude a daily habit b) Decrease life satisfaction c) Increase negative emotions d) None of the above

5. Expressing gratitude to others can lead to: a) Improved relationship quality b) Reduced feelings of connection and satisfaction c) Decreased sense of gratitude d) None of the above

(Answers: 1d, 2False, 3b, 4a, 5a)

References

- Emmons, R. A., & McCullough, M. E. (2003). Counting blessings versus burdens: An experimental investigation of gratitude and subjective well-being in daily life. Journal of Personality and Social Psychology, 84(2), 377.

- Seligman, M. E., Steen, T. A., Park, N., & Peterson, C. (2005). Positive psychology progress: empirical validation of interventions. American psychologist, 60(5), 410.

- Kabat-Zinn, J. (1994). Wherever you go, there you are: Mindfulness meditation in everyday life. Hyperion.

- Algoe, S. B., Gable, S. L., & Maisel, N. C. (2010). It's the little things: Everyday gratitude as a booster shot for romantic relationships. Personal Relationships, 17(2), 217-233.

- Wood, A. M., Joseph, S., Lloyd, J., & Atkins, S. (2009). Gratitude influences sleep through the mechanism of pre-sleep cognitions. Journal of Psychosomatic Research, 66(1), 43-48.

- Lambert, N. M., Fincham, F. D., & Stillman, T. F. (2012). Gratitude and depressive symptoms: the role of positive reframing and positive emotion. Cognition and Emotion, 26(4), 615-633.

- Algoe, S. B. (2012). Find, remind, and bind: The functions of gratitude in everyday relationships. Social and Personality Psychology Compass, 6(6), 455-469.

Lesson 8

Leveraging Gratitude During Difficult Times

Life isn't always easy; we all face hardships, losses, and periods of adversity. However, even in these difficult times, the practice of gratitude can serve as a beacon of light, helping us navigate through the storm. In this lesson, we'll delve into the science of gratitude during times of adversity, understand its protective and healing effects, and learn ways to cultivate it even when times are hard.

The Protective Role of Gratitude

Life is full of difficulties, and everyone experiences adversity at some point. During these challenging times, gratitude can play a crucial role in our emotional wellbeing.

In two studies of populations facing serious personal difficulties (patients with neuromuscular disease and people recovering from substance misuse), Wood, Joseph, and Linley (2007) found that gratitude correlated with lower stress and depression. The researchers suggested that gratitude might give people a positive perspective from which to view negative life events.

The practice of gratitude has been associated with resilience, a key factor in overcoming adversity and building mental strength. In a study conducted by Kleiman et al. (2013), individuals who expressed gratitude showed a greater ability to cope with traumatic life events and exhibited higher resilience.

Killen and Macaskill (2015) found that gratitude was related to greater resilience among adolescents after the Christchurch earthquakes, suggesting that gratitude may play a significant role in recovery after traumatic events.

In a study conducted with Vietnam War Veterans, Kashdan et al. (2006) reported that those veterans who reported more gratitude experienced lower rates of Post-Traumatic Stress Disorder (PTSD). The researchers suggested that the positive emotionality associated with gratitude could provide a buffer against the severe anxiety associated with PTSD.

Mechanisms of the protective aspect of gratitude:

1. **Cognitive Coping:** Gratitude encourages us to focus on the positive aspects of our lives, which can help in reframing negative or stressful situations (Lambert et al., 2009). This shift in perspective allows us to find meaning and cultivate a sense of purpose during challenging times.

2. **Emotional Coping:** Gratitude promotes positive emotions such as joy, contentment, and love, which can counterbalance the negative emotions that often accompany adversity (Emmons & McCullough, 2003). This emotional counterweight can improve our mood and overall psychological wellbeing.

Unpacking the Benefits: How Does Gratitude Help?

Now, let's look at how gratitude might provide these benefits during challenging times.

- Positive Reframing: Gratitude helps us to see our circumstances in a new light. Even in the face of adversity, there are often aspects of our lives for which we can be grateful. By focusing on these positive elements, we can reframe our experiences in a way that makes them easier to bear.

- Emotional Resilience: Gratitude can increase our emotional resilience, helping us bounce back from negative events more quickly and effectively. By acknowledging the good in our lives, we can balance out the impact of the bad, reducing our emotional reactions to negative events.

- Strengthening Relationships: Gratitude can strengthen our relationships, providing us with a support system during challenging times. When we express gratitude to others, it can deepen our connections, making others more likely to provide emotional support when we need it.

- Boosting Positive Emotions: Even in difficult times, gratitude can boost positive emotions. Research has shown that positive emotions can help us cope with stress and adversity, making gratitude a valuable tool in difficult times.

Gratitude and Trauma Recovery

Experiencing traumatic events can lead to intense negative emotions and even post-traumatic stress disorder (PTSD). However, studies suggest that gratitude may play a role in trauma recovery.

In a study by Vernon et al. (2009), trauma survivors who expressed gratitude experienced fewer PTSD symptoms. Their study also showed a link between gratitude and posttraumatic growth, a psychological transformation resulting in better functioning after trauma. This suggests that gratitude can be a vital tool in trauma recovery and posttraumatic growth, offering a ray of hope in our darkest times.

Gratitude as a Buffer Against Stress

Life's difficulties often bring stress, but gratitude can serve as a buffer against this common mental health concern. In their research, Wood et al. (2008) found that gratitude was associated with lower stress and depression levels. They theorized grateful people are more likely to perceive social support, decrease their negative appraisals of stressful events, and effectively cope with stress.

Gratitude and Physical Health

In times of physical illness or when dealing with chronic pain, cultivating gratitude can have a remarkable effect. A study conducted by Jackowska, Brown, Ronaldson, and Steptoe (2016) demonstrated that patients who maintained a grateful outlook experienced less severe disease symptoms and maintained better physical health than those who didn't.

The concept is that focusing on positive emotions, such as gratitude, can lead to a healthier lifestyle and better immune responses. It encourages behaviors like regular exercise, a balanced diet, and adequate sleep, and all these factors contribute to better health.

Gratitude and Grief

Gratitude can also be a significant source of resilience during periods of loss and grief. According to a study by Linley and Joseph (2004), individuals who found benefits and showed gratitude during bereavement reported better adaptation and less distress.

While it might be challenging to be grateful during such periods, recognizing small moments of reprieve or remembering the positive memories of the lost loved one can facilitate the grieving process.

Increasing Awareness of Complaining

While gratitude encourages a focus on the positive, it's essential to recognize and address its counterpart: complaining. Complaining, while natural, can sometimes hinder our ability to see and appreciate the good in our lives. By increasing our awareness of complaining, we can make a more conscious effort to shift towards gratitude.

Effects of Complaining:

1. Mood Influencer: Regular complaining can foster a negative mindset, which affects our mood and overall outlook on life.

2. Relationship Impact: Constant complaints can strain relationships, making interactions less enjoyable for both parties.

3. Missed Opportunities: When we're focused on what's wrong, we might overlook the good or miss opportunities to find solutions to our challenges.

Gratitude as a Pathway to Growth

Experiencing adversity can provide an opportunity for personal growth, and gratitude can be the key to unlocking this potential. In post-traumatic growth, people find positive change and new life possibilities after trauma.

Research by Tedeschi and Calhoun (2004) suggests that gratitude can help individuals appreciate life more, recognize alternative paths for their lives, improve their personal strength, and enhance their relationships, even in the aftermath of traumatic events. Cultivating gratitude can, therefore, lead to the discovery of a deeper sense of purpose and a greater appreciation of life's value, despite the hardships endured.

Gratitude serves as more than just a tool for enhancing our well-being during good times; By helping us reframe our experiences, boosting our resilience, strengthening our relationships, and promoting positive emotions, gratitude can provide a much-needed light in the darkness.

Exercise: Gratitude Journaling During Tough Times

Despite the apparent benefits of gratitude during hard times, it's challenging to feel thankful when you're struggling. To help cultivate gratitude during adversity, try this exercise: Gratitude Journaling During Tough Times.

Each day, find at least three things for which you're grateful. They can be simple, like a warm cup of coffee, or more profound, like love from your family. Reflect on these positive aspects and write them down.

Remember, it's okay if you struggle at first - the aim isn't to deny or ignore your hardships, but to allow yourself to recognize that even in tough times, good things can exist.

Interactive Activity: Complaint Awareness Jar

Objective: To increase awareness of how often you complain and encourage a shift towards gratitude.

Materials: A jar, a pack of small beads or coins, a notepad, and a pen.

Steps:

1. Setup: Place the jar in a location you frequent daily, such as your living room or office desk. Keep the beads or coins and the notepad nearby.

2. Daily Practice: Every time you catch yourself complaining, drop a bead or coin into the jar. It doesn't matter if the complaint is big or small; the goal is to become more aware.

3. Reflection: At the end of each day, count the number of beads or coins in the jar and jot down the total in the notepad. Take a moment to reflect on your complaints. Were they necessary? Could you have approached the situation differently?

4. Weekly Review: At the end of the week, review your daily counts. Do you notice any patterns or improvements?

5. Shift to Gratitude: For every complaint you recorded, try to think of one thing you're grateful for. This practice will help balance out the negatives with positives.

Tip: As you become more aware of your complaints, challenge yourself to reduce the number of beads or coins you add to the jar each day. Over time, you'll likely complain less and appreciating more.

Quiz

1. What role does gratitude play during challenging times?

2. Discuss how gratitude can aid in trauma recovery.

3. How can gratitude act as a buffer against stress?

4. Describe the Gratitude Journaling During Tough Times exercise.

Extended Quiz

1. How can gratitude influence physical health during challenging times?

2. Discuss the role of gratitude in the process of grief.

3. Explain the concept of post-traumatic growth and the role of gratitude in it.

4. Describe the detrimental effects of complaining.

References

- Kleiman, E. M., Adams, L. M., Kashdan, T. B., & Riskind, J. H. (2013). Gratitude and grit indirectly reduce risk of suicidal ideations by enhancing meaning in life: Evidence for a mediated moderation model. Journal of Research in Personality, 47(5), 539-546.

- Lambert, N. M., Clark, M. S., Durtschi, J., Fincham, F. D., & Graham, S. M. (2009). Benefits of Expressing Gratitude: Expressing Gratitude to a Partner Changes One's View of the Relationship. Psychological Science, 20(4), 574–580.

- Emmons, R. A., & McCullough, M. E. (2003). Counting blessings versus burdens: an experimental investigation of gratitude and subjective well-being in daily life. Journal of personality and social psychology, 84(2), 377-389.

- Vernon, L. L., Dillon, J. M., & Steiner, A. R. W. (2009). Proactive coping, gratitude, and posttraumatic stress disorder in college women. Anxiety, Stress, & Coping, 22(1), 117–127.

- Wood, A. M., Joseph, S., & Maltby, J. (2008). Gratitude predicts psychological well-being above the Big Five facets. Personality and Individual Differences, 46(4), 443–447.

- Jackowska, M., Brown, J., Ronaldson, A., & Steptoe, A. (2016). The impact of a brief gratitude intervention on subjective well-being, biology and sleep. Journal of Health Psychology, 21(10), 2207-2217.

- Linley, P. A., & Joseph, S. (2004). Positive change following trauma and adversity: A review. Journal of Traumatic Stress, 17(1), 11-21.

- Tedeschi, R. G., & Calhoun, L. G. (2004). Posttraumatic Growth: Conceptual Foundations and Empirical Evidence. Psychological Inquiry, 15(1), 1–18.

Gratitude for Personal Growth

In this lesson, we'll explore the fundamental role of gratitude in promoting personal growth. We'll delve into the empirical evidence that highlights the transformative power of gratitude on our personal development journey and provide practical exercises to cultivate this beneficial attitude.

The Impact of Gratitude on Personal Growth

Personal growth is the process of self-improvement, encompassing development in personal skills, knowledge, and self-awareness. It's a lifelong journey of learning and transformation, and gratitude can play a crucial part in this process.

According to research, gratitude doesn't just make us feel good; it encourages us to become better versions of ourselves. It enhances our self-esteem, improves our relationships, and pushes us towards our goals.

A study conducted by Kashdan, Uswatte, and Julian (2006) showed that gratitude encourages personal growth by making us appreciate the value of present moments. This mindful appreciation enables us to learn from our experiences and move forward in a more positive and informed manner.

Gratitude and Self-Esteem

Research shows a significant positive effect of gratitude on self-esteem, a vital component of personal growth. Gratitude helps us to appreciate others' accomplishments without feeling threatened or inadequate, fostering a healthier self-image.

Research by Chen, Chen, Kee, and Tsai (2009) suggested that individuals who practice gratitude regularly have higher self-esteem than those who don't. When we focus on what we have, rather than what we lack, we develop a more positive self-image, which forms the basis for personal growth.

Gratitude and Goal Achievement

Goal achievement is an important part of personal growth, and gratitude can help us reach our goals more effectively. By acknowledging our accomplishments and celebrating the journey, gratitude can boost our motivation and commitment to personal development goals.

In a study by Emmons and McCullough (2003), those who kept gratitude journals were more likely to make progress towards their personal goals. By regularly expressing gratitude, we can remain focused, motivated, and appreciative of our growth process.

The Role of Gratitude in Resilience Building

Resilience, the capacity to bounce back from adversity, is another key element of personal growth. And gratitude plays an essential role in building this resilience.

Psychological resilience enables individuals to navigate through adversities and effectively cope with life's inevitable challenges. It is the ability to 'bounce back' and adapt following setbacks. By focusing on the positive aspects of life, gratitude allows us to see beyond our current problems and view these issues within a broader context of life's overall goodness. This change of perspective can significantly increase our resilience.

In their 2008 study, Wood, Maltby, Stewart, and Joseph discovered a strong correlation between gratitude and resilience in the face of adversity. Those who reported higher levels of gratitude showed greater resilience and less stress and depression.

Gratitude, Self-Awareness, and Emotional Intelligence

Gratitude doesn't just make us happier; it makes us smarter about understanding our own emotions and those of others. This boosts our emotional intelligence and promotes our personal growth.

Gratitude helps us become more aware of our own experiences, reducing our focus on negatives and enhancing our overall self-awareness. This self-awareness is a cornerstone of emotional intelligence and is critical in understanding our own emotions, what causes them, and how they impact our thoughts and behaviors.

By promoting empathy and perspective-taking, gratitude allows us to better understand and respond to other people's emotions. This social aspect of emotional intelligence is crucial for building strong, supportive relationships that can foster personal growth.

Gratitude and Optimism

Optimism is another essential component of personal growth. By fostering a positive outlook, we can approach our personal development journey with enthusiasm and hope.

Gratitude is a powerful catalyst for optimism. By routinely acknowledging the good in our lives, we can cultivate a more positive outlook. The focus shifts from what's going wrong to the wealth of things going right.

Research by Wood, Joseph, and Maltby (2009) revealed that gratitude was a significant predictor of optimism, suggesting that gratitude practices can effectively enhance our positive outlook and contribute to our personal growth.

Exercise: Gratitude Letter for Personal Growth

This exercise involves writing a letter to yourself. Reflect on your personal growth journey so far. Acknowledge the progress you've made, express gratitude for the lessons learned, the challenges overcome, and the strength you have gained. Recognize the people who supported you along the way. Don't rush this process; take the time to genuinely express your gratitude.

Extended Exercise: The Future Gratitude Letter

Besides writing a gratitude letter for your personal growth so far, consider writing a letter to your future self, expressing gratitude for the growth you expect. This can help you clarify your personal growth goals and nurture an optimistic outlook for your growth journey.

Quiz

1. Explain how gratitude can affect personal growth.

2. Discuss the role of gratitude in enhancing self-esteem.

3. How does gratitude facilitate goal achievement?

4. Describe the Gratitude Letter for Personal Growth exercise.

Extended Quiz

1. How does gratitude contribute to resilience building?

2. Discuss the relationship between gratitude and self-awareness.

3. How does gratitude influence our level of optimism?

4. Describe the Future Gratitude Letter exercise and its benefits.

References

- Kashdan, T. B., Uswatte, G., & Julian, T. (2006). Gratitude and hedonic and eudaimonic well-being in Vietnam war veterans. Behaviour Research and Therapy, 44(2), 177–199.

- Chen, L. H., Chen, M. Y., Kee, Y. H., & Tsai, Y. M. (2009). Validation of the Gratitude Questionnaire (GQ) in Taiwanese undergraduate students. Journal of Happiness Studies, 10(6), 655–664.

- Emmons, R. A., & McCullough, M. E. (2003). Counting blessings versus burdens: an experimental investigation of gratitude and subjective well-being in daily life. Journal of Personality and Social Psychology, 84(2), 377–389.

- Wood, A. M., Maltby, J., Stewart, N., & Joseph, S. (2008). A social-cognitive model of trait and state levels of gratitude. Emotion, 8(2), 281-290.

- Wood, A. M., Joseph, S., & Maltby, J. (2009). Gratitude predicts psychological well-being above the Big Five facets. Personality and Individual Differences, 46(4), 443–447.

Lesson 10

Gratitude in Context - The Significance of Authenticity

Introduction

While the previous lessons have explained the myriad benefits of gratitude, it's essential to approach this powerful concept and emotion with a holistic view. We can use gratitude as one component of well-being, and understanding its proper context is vital. This lesson emphasizes the importance of authenticity in feeling gratitude and sheds light on the intricacies of the scientific studies in this domain.

1. Gratitude: A Piece of the Puzzle

- **Holistic Well-being:** Total wellness isn't only physical but encompasses all aspects of an individual, including behavioral, emotional, social, spiritual, and psychological dimensions. While gratitude can significantly affect overall well-being, other elements like nutrition, exercise, meditation, and social connections also play pivotal roles. Therefore, gratitude is a tool, not a panacea.

- **Contextual Relevance:** The positive effects of gratitude may vary based on individual circumstances. For instance, someone going through severe depression or trauma might benefit from various interventions, with gratitude being just one of them.

2. Authenticity Matters

- **Sincerity:** True benefits emerge when gratitude is genuine. Feigned or artificial gratitude might not only be ineffective, but could also be counterproductive. A person might feel pressure or guilt for not feeling grateful, leading to added emotional distress.

- **Individual Differences:** It's crucial to recognize that everyone has their rhythm of experiencing emotions. Pressuring oneself or others to feel grateful in every situation can be disingenuous.

3. Not as Black and White

- **Designing Studies:** The subjective nature of gratitude poses challenges in designing and conceptualizing studies. Quantifying such an emotion accurately requires nuanced methodologies.

- **Varied Results:** Not all research on gratitude reports positive outcomes. Researchers in some studies found negligible effects, particularly if gratitude was forced or became a source of stress.

- **Replicability Crisis:** Some findings in psychological science, including those related to gratitude, haven't been reproducible. This doesn't negate the benefits of gratitude, but underlines the need for robust research methodologies. This is also not unusual in scientific studies on humans. It's very difficult in human studies to isolate variables in a study.

4. **When Gratitude Doesn't Work**

- **Overemphasis:** Overemphasizing gratitude in situations that demand other emotional responses (like grief, anger, or sadness) can invalidate and harmful.

- **Toxic Positivity:** Gratitude shouldn't be used to suppress or dismiss genuine negative feelings. This phenomenon, called toxic positivity, can lead to emotional repression.

- **One Size Doesn't Fit All:** Just as medicines have varied effects on individuals, gratitude interventions may not work universally. It's essential to tailor well-being tools to individual needs.

Incorporating gratitude as part of a comprehensive approach to mental health: A Potent but Balanced Approach

Mental health is a complex interplay of biological, psychological, and social factors. In recent years, the field of psychology has expanded its lens to look beyond just symptom reduction, focusing also on holistic well-being. One practice that has received significant attention is gratitude. While it isn't a cure-all, gratitude has emerged as a powerful tool in holistic mental health regimens.

Gratitude, simply put, is the acknowledgment of the good in life. Whether it's appreciating a kind act, recognizing our personal strengths, or savoring nature's beauty, gratitude has a way of focusing the mind on the positive.

As we have discussed at length, scientific studies on gratitude have shown its potential benefits, such as:

- Improved mood and reduced depressive symptoms.

- Increased life satisfaction.

- Strengthened resilience.

- Enhanced relationships.

A study published in the Journal of Personality and Social Psychology found that regularly journaling about gratitude could lead to increased optimism and improved well-being. Another research in Applied Psychology: Health and Well-Being noted that gratitude interventions could be especially beneficial for individuals with mental health issues.

Gratitude in Holistic Mental Health Treatment

Conventional Western medicine, also called allopathic medicine, focuses almost exclusively on the physical. It's only recently that there has been any emphasis on mental health and on social determinants of health. Practitioners largely ignore the behavioral, emotional, social, cultural, and spiritual aspects of an individual. Admittedly, many of the most common issues, such as headaches, belly pain, diffuse body pain, and fatigue, are "stress" related issues. Regardless, we treat the physical symptom with pharmaceuticals or sometimes even procedures and not treat the foundational causes, mostly because it's easier. Newer forms of therapy, such as those used in counseling or positive psychology, attempt to address these issues at a more foundational level. Here's how gratitude fits into this paradigm:

1. **Cognitive Re-framing:** Negative thought patterns are common in conditions like depression and anxiety. Gratitude practices can serve as a cognitive tool to help individuals shift their focus from what's lacking or negative to what's abundant and positive in their lives.

2. **Enhancing Mindfulness:** Mindfulness is the practice of staying present. When combined with gratitude, individuals learn not only to be present but also to find moments of appreciation in the now, be it in a breath, a sound, or a memory.

3. **Body and Spirit:** Gratitude can lead to reduced stress levels, which has physiological benefits, such as lower blood pressure and improved immune function. Spiritually, gratitude often plays a role in grounding, providing a sense of connection to something bigger—whether it's nature, humanity, or a higher power.

A Note of Caution

While gratitude has its merits, it's crucial to approach it with balance:

- **Gratitude isn't a Panacea:** It's essential to remember that gratitude isn't a replacement for comprehensive mental health treatments, such as professional counseling or medication. It's an adjunct, another tool in the toolbox.

- **The Danger of Forced Gratitude:** Genuine gratitude has its benefits, but forced or feigned gratitude can be counterproductive. Individuals should never feel pressured into gratitude, especially during challenging times. Please see the "Recommended Reading" below.

- Gratitude has to be authentic to be effective. I believe that's one issue of many that makes research studies challenging.

Importantly, I have found that mostly when someone is ready to let go of a hurt or a held victim scenario, they can find something they can be grateful for within it. Often it starts with one small thing. Later it grows to bigger ones. It doesn't happen until someone is ready. In our training, we emphasize holding onto hurts causes you pain and suffering, not the other person. You look to let it go for you, not for the one who "victimized" you. Even if you forgive them, you do it for you. We focus on this in the self-awareness portion of our program.

Incorporating gratitude into your life on a regular daily basis.

1. **Gratitude Journaling:** Setting aside a few minutes daily to write about moments or things one is grateful for can gradually shift mindset.

2. **Gratitude Meditation:** Combining gratitude with meditation can enhance both practices, grounding individuals in the present moment.

3. **Gratitude Reminders:** Using notes, alarms, or apps to sprinkle moments of gratitude throughout the day can help reinforce the practice. Finding gratitude for small, everyday, common occurrences or events. I call these "Gratitude Bites". I offer daily gratitude emails or texts as an option.

Conclusion

Gratitude, when genuine and practiced mindfully, can be a transformative emotion. However, it's essential to understand its place in the larger wellness paradigm. It's one of many tools we possess in the pursuit of a meaningful, joyful, and healthy life. As with any tool, it's most effective when used appropriately and with other well-being strategies.

Assignment for Next Session: Reflect on a situation where gratitude felt forced or inauthentic. How did it make you feel? Contrast it with an instance of genuine gratitude. How were the experiences different, and what can you learn from them?

Recommended Readings:

- "How Gratitude Can Harm Mental Health—and Ways Around It" by Amanda Ann Gregory, LCPC.

- "The Replicability Crisis in Psychological Science" by Dr. Farid Anvari.

- "Toxic Positivity" Psychology Today

Exercise: Authentic Gratitude Journaling

Objective: This exercise helps you differentiate between moments of genuine gratitude and times when gratitude might feel forced. It promotes self-awareness and a more profound understanding of your feelings.

Duration: 15-20 minutes daily for one week.

Materials: A notebook or journal, a pen.

Instructions:

1. **Setting the Scene:** Choose a quiet location, free from distractions. Sit comfortably and take a few deep breaths to center yourself.

2. **Recalling the Day:** Think about your day from the moment you woke until the present. Recollect significant events, interactions, feelings, and thoughts.

3. **Journaling:**

    - **Genuine Gratitude:** Write three moments or things from the day for which you felt genuine gratitude, no matter how big or small. Describe the situation and detail how it made you feel. For example, "I felt genuinely grateful when my colleague offered to help with my workload today. It made me feel supported and valued."

    - **Forced Gratitude:** Reflect on any moment during the day where you felt you should be grateful, but weren't genuinely feeling it. Describe the situation and explore why you felt the gratitude might be inauthentic. For example, "I was told to feel grateful for the challenging feedback from my manager because it's 'for my growth,' but I felt more hurt and unrecognized than grateful."

4. **Reflection:** After journaling, take a few minutes to read your entries. Reflect on the differences between genuine and forced gratitude. How do they impact your well-being, mood, and perception of events?

5. **Consistency:** Repeat this exercise daily for a week.

Follow-up:

At the end of the week, review your journal entries. Look for patterns in your experiences. This review will provide insights into situations that naturally elicit gratitude and those where gratitude feels imposed. It's a way of understanding your emotional responses better and promotes self-awareness.

Essential Tip: Remember, there's no judgment in this exercise. It's a personal tool to help you understand your relationship with gratitude. It's perfectly okay not to feel grateful all the time; the aim is to recognize and appreciate authentic moments of gratitude in your life.

Quiz: Authentic Gratitude

1. Which of the following describes the best approach to gratitude? a) Feeling grateful in every situation, no matter what. b) Expressing gratitude only when it feels genuine. c) Using gratitude to suppress negative emotions. d) Making others always express gratitude.

Answer: b) Expressing gratitude only when it feels genuine.

2. In which situation is emphasizing gratitude likely harmful? a) Celebrating a birthday. b) Grieving a loss. c) Enjoying a meal. d) Spending time with loved ones.

Answer: b) Grieving a loss.

3. What challenge is common in designing scientific studies on gratitude? a) The emotion is easily quantifiable. b) Gratitude is universally experienced the same way. c) The subjective nature of gratitude. d) Everyone shows gratitude outwardly.

Answer: c) The subjective nature of gratitude.

References:

1. Emmons, R. A., & McCullough, M. E. (2003). Counting blessings versus burdens: An experimental investigation of gratitude and subjective well-being in daily life. *Journal of Personality and Social Psychology,* 84(2), 377.

2. Watkins, P. C., Woodward, K., Stone, T., & Kolts, R. L. (2003). Gratitude and happiness: Development of a measure of gratitude and relationships with subjective well-being. *Social Behavior and Personality: an international journal,* 31(5), 431-452.

3. Fredrickson, B. L. (2001). The role of positive emotions in positive psychology: The broaden-and-build theory of positive emotions. *American psychologist,* 56(3), 218.

4. Tugade, M. M., & Fredrickson, B. L. (2004). Resilient individuals use positive emotions to bounce back from negative emotional experiences. *Journal of Personality and Social Psychology,* 86(2), 320.

5. Burton, C. M., & King, L. A. (2004). The health benefits of writing about intensely positive experiences. *Journal of Research in Personality,* 38(2), 150-163.

6. Neff, K. D. (2011). Self-compassion, self-esteem, and well-being. *Social and personality psychology compass,* 5(1), 1-12. (This provides insights on the dangers of toxic positivity.)

Remember, these exercises, quizzes, and references are tools to enhance your understanding and are not definitive answers to the vast, intricate world of gratitude and positive psychology.